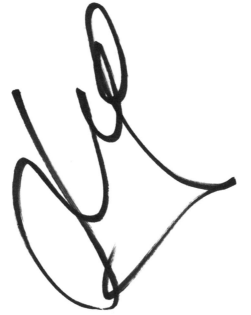

# THE NATURAL WAY
## TO
# BEAT DIABETES

Prevention®

# The
# NATURAL WAY
## to
# BEAT
# DIABETES

A TOTAL LIFE PLAN TO HELP YOU

Lose Weight,
Gain Energy, *and*
Take Control of Your Health

**Spencer Nadolsky, DO,** and Lou Schuler

RODALE.

© 2017 by Rodale Inc.

Photographs by Mitch Mandel/Rodale Images

Book design by Christina Gaugler

Library of Congress Cataloging-in-Publication Data is on file with the publisher.

ISBN 978-1-62336-868-5

2   4   6   8   10   9   7   5   3   1   hardcover

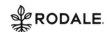

We inspire health, healing, happiness, and love in the world.
Starting with you.

# Contents

# Part Four: TREATMENT AND RECOVERY

# What Does "Natural" Even Mean?

**I'M A DOCTOR WHO SPECIALIZES** in obesity and diabetes. Patients don't come to me until they have a problem in one of those areas, and usually both. Sometimes they come to my office with dread, knowing I'm going to tell them something they already suspect but don't want to confirm. Sometimes it's with hope that I can offer a solution their last doctor—or multiple doctors—couldn't, wouldn't, or simply didn't provide.

My practice is driven by two urgent questions.

- How can I help patients get better?

- What can I say, do, or prescribe that will be more effective than what they've already heard, done, or taken?

The treatment I recommend may or may not include drugs. But there's a 100 percent chance it will include exercise, diet, and lifestyle management. In my experience, in my practice, and in my very firm opinion, nothing works better for my patients than the measures they take to help themselves.

First comes diet. Changing even a few things around, making *somewhat* better choices *most* of the time, is the most effective intervention. Close behind is exercise. A patient who goes from sedentary to regularly active is healthier than she was before and feels better about herself. It's simultaneously powerful and empowering. To show how important it is, I'll sometimes go to the gym with my patients to coach them on key exercises and take them through a workout. Third is lifestyle management. It starts with getting more sleep, and better sleep, but it also means keeping a regular, predictable schedule—going to bed and waking up at about the same time every day.

If more people simply did those three things, I'd prescribe a lot less medicine. For some patients I mean that literally—with diet, exercise, and lifestyle improvements, they need less medicine than they did when they walked into my office for the first time. For others, it means no medicine at all. Either they manage their diabetes so well they no longer need the drugs they currently take, or they reverse the condition before I write the first script.

Which brings me to the elephant in the room—or, at least, the gigantic pachyderm in the title of this book.

## OUR UNNATURAL WORLD

Few words in the English language are used as often as "natural," with so little meaning. (Although "unsubscribe" comes pretty close.) It's a great word for marketers because it implies something slightly different to everyone they reach, depending on their values and fears.

For one person a "natural" product is made entirely from things that are found in nature, implying that humans simply assembled the parts or ingredients. For another it might suggest a product is safe. Just about everybody understands that the opposite of "natural" is "unnatural." So even if we don't stop to think what exactly is "natural" about a bar of soap or a frozen dinner, we know not to be afraid of it.

There is almost nothing natural about diabetes. The overwhelming majority of cases are caused by our unnatural environment, which provides too much food and requires too little exercise. An unnatural disease calls for unnatural measures, including frequent blood tests and powerful medicines. Because I'm a physician, it's my job to perform those tests and prescribe those medicines.

Those invasive and, too often, *expensive* measures can be minimized by changing your diet, activity level, and sleep habits. You can call the changes "natural" if you want, or use a fancier euphemism like "lifestyle modification." But the reality is, if you're reading a book with "diabetes" in the title, all these choices will seem anything but natural.

It's human nature to eat food when it's right there in front of us. It's human nature to preserve our energy and move only when we have to. It's human nature to enjoy being entertained, even if that entertainment comes out of a TV or smartphone screen and disrupts our sleep. What I describe as the "natural" way to beat diabetes is to disrupt the comfortable patterns of your life and make choices that will be pretty challenging at first.

I do it because it works. I have yet to prescribe a drug as powerful as exercise. Nothing we've invented comes close to what we were born with: bodies that thrive on movement. A better diet will not only reduce your weight, but also your risk of diabetes, if you don't yet have it, or the severity of it if you do. Better sleep makes it much easier to manage your appetite and to get more exercise.

These three tools come with substantial benefits and no serious risks (as long as you're careful to look both ways before crossing the street on your daily walks). You don't have to worry about adverse reactions. Unlike most drugs, lifestyle tools have additive effects. Each improves the results of the others.

Over these pages you'll see the evidence for everything I just said, including both scientific data and my own experiences with patients. You'll also find a lot of information about the medicines I prescribe for managing diabetes. I'll highlight the most important and commonly used drugs, describe what they are and how they work, and explain when I do or don't use them. If you're already taking one or more of those drugs, I hope your doctor has explained all this. But whether he has or hasn't, the information is there for you.

# BEYOND THE BASICS

What I've described so far probably sounds familiar: "Eat less, move more." Chances are you've heard those words, in that order, from your doctor, your family, your coworkers, and even random strangers. (We do live in rude times.) They come at you not as well-meaning advice, but as mean-spirited judgment. I'm on record as saying that "eat less, move more," in isolation, is terrible advice; it's akin to telling a depressed person to "cheer up" or counseling an alcoholic to drink less. If it actually worked, you wouldn't be reading this book because I wouldn't have written it.

Sure, you can say that's what my advice boils down to, and it would be accurate enough. But it wouldn't come close to describing my message. I'm going to show you, literally from the first step, *how* to move more. I'm going to talk about the best times to move, the best systems of exercise, and the best ways to make meaningful, measurable progress.

Same with the "eat less" side of the equation. My colleagues and I don't get much nutrition training in medical school, and my patients have told me about doctors who measure your height and weight, tell you you're fat, and send you out the door with a brochure detailing which vegetables you should eat more of. My program starts with the simplest, most painless changes to your eating habits, the ones that allow you to eat less without feeling especially deprived. From there I'll show you how to build a sustainable diet that helps you lose weight, lower your blood sugar, and minimize hunger.

That's how you'll beat diabetes: not with some drugs and a four-word phrase that fits on a bumper sticker, but with a progressive, systematic, lifestyle-focused approach. It may not be entirely "natural," but in these overstuffed times we live in, what is?

# PART ONE

# How Did This Happen to Me?

## CHAPTER 1

# "Another Patient Went Off Insulin Today"

**JASON HADN'T BEEN TO A DOCTOR** in many years before he came to see me. At 45, he weighed 255 pounds, with a 43-inch waist. He told me he had been experiencing dizziness and was urinating like a racehorse, as if his bladder had doubled in size and filled twice as fast.

I checked his blood sugar. Anything more than 200 milligrams per deciliter suggests diabetes. Jason's was close to 400. It was one of the highest random blood sugar tests I've ever seen. My immediate fear was that he was in a state called diabetic ketoacidosis, or DKA, a medical condition that's often preceded by the words "potentially fatal." I sent him directly to the emergency room.

Jason's story, which I'll return to in a moment, is probably different from yours. You may be a different gender, older or younger, bigger or smaller. Maybe your doctor gave you the news about your diabetes yesterday, and you're still in shock. Or perhaps you've been dealing with it for years. It's also possible you've been told you have prediabetes, which means you have all the warning signs but don't yet have the disease.

One thing you probably have in common with Jason: You're scared, and you should be. *Diabetes* is four syllables of fear. I know because I've seen that initial reaction too many times, in too many patients. The word conjures up thoughts of a lifetime on heavy-duty medications, culminating in blindness and amputations. And for some people, unfortunately, that is the way it goes down. But it's not inevitable.

About 95 percent of people with diabetes have type 2, which, in the majority of cases, is a disease of excess: too much food, with too little exercise, for too many years. For some of my patients, like Jason, the diagnosis isn't really a surprise. Anyone who searches online for "blurred vision" and/or "excessive urination" will get a free diagnosis from Dr. Google. For many others, it's a shock to hear the news. You can't feel high blood sugar or insulin resistance. But for almost everyone with type 2 diabetes, the disease is a progression of steadily increasing weight coinciding with rising blood sugar, triglycerides, blood pressure, and many other markers of poor health and high risk not just for diabetes, but for a long list of even scarier diseases.

That's why the best treatment is also a progression, only this time in the opposite direction. If diabetes is a disease of excess nutrition, the solution *has* to begin with the opposite. You don't need to make huge cuts. In fact, as I'll explain in Part Two, you may not even notice the first calories you delete, much less miss them. But there's no getting around the need to eat less food and to make better choices in your diet.

The same applies to exercise. If too little movement—combined with too many hours in front of your computer or TV, or behind the wheel of your car, or stretched out on the couch—created the perfect environment for diabetes, then moving more is part of the solution. The goal isn't to turn you into a marathoner or mountain climber or bodybuilder. If you *want* to do any of those things, great; this book could very well get you started down that path. But for now, we'll start where you are, with the goal of doing just a little more. If you're not doing anything, a little more than zero is pretty easy, as you'll see in Chapter 4.

We'll get into the complexities of lifestyle change as we go along, including one that makes the others possible: sleep. A diabetes-reversing lifestyle begins and ends with a good night's sleep, something that many of my patients struggle with. Deep, restorative slumber gives you the mental energy to stick with your diet plan and the physical energy to exercise. It's the difference between hating your new life and reveling in it.

## DIABETES: THE BASICS

- Diabetes is a disruption in the way your body processes glucose, also known as blood sugar.

- About 5 percent of all patients have type 1 diabetes, in which the pancreas doesn't make enough insulin, the hormone responsible for pushing glucose into your cells, where it can be used for energy.

- About 95 percent of patients have type 2, in which your body becomes resistant to insulin. Most of the time, your pancreas initially responds by making more of it. But eventually it slows down or stops altogether, making you dependent on medical insulin.

- As of 2012, an estimated 29.1 million Americans had diabetes. Another 86 million had prediabetes, which means they have elevated blood glucose but aren't yet considered diabetic. Combined they make up more than a third of the US population.

- About 1.4 million Americans receive a diabetes diagnosis every year.

- Diabetes is the seventh leading cause of death in the United States and also contributes to many deaths from cardiovascular disease and other conditions.

- The annual cost of treating diabetes in the United States is an estimated $245 billion. That includes $176 billion in medical expenses and $69 billion in reduced productivity.

- Globally, experts believe 422 million people have diabetes, and that it kills about 1.5 million a year. An additional 2.2 million annual deaths from heart, kidney, and lung diseases are attributed to high blood glucose.

Jason is a perfect example. As I guessed the first time he came to my office, a 45-year-old guy with a 43-inch waist wasn't wearing out the equipment at the local Planet Fitness. I saw him again a week later. This time he had an ambitious goal. The doctors at the hospital had prescribed a relatively high dose of insulin to help reduce his blood sugar, and he wanted to get off it as soon as possible.

I explained what he was up against as tactfully as I could. But there's really no sugarcoating the message. His fondness for fast food, and aversion to exercise, had nearly killed him. The high insulin dose had saved his life by bringing his blood sugar down. It was now close to the normal range. I agreed to cut his dose in half, but with two conditions: He had to eat a lot less junk food and get a little more exercise. I also prescribed two other medications, with the understanding that if he followed the program, I'd be able to reduce those as well. (I'll go into much more detail about medicine in Part Four.)

To my surprise, and perhaps to his, he didn't just follow my advice. He *exceeded* it by walking 2 hours a day. When I saw him a week later, his fasting blood sugar was below 100—normal for a healthy, nondiabetic adult—and he'd already lost a few pounds. I cut his insulin down to the lowest possible dose. A week after that, his blood sugar was still in the healthy range, so I took him off insulin altogether.

Jason came to see me once a month. Each time, he was 5 to 10 pounds lighter. In less than a year he was down to 200 pounds, a loss of 22 percent of his initial body weight, with a 36-inch waist. His clothes were falling off. He had a bounce in his step that wasn't there before. On one visit he marveled at how much energy he had; to him, it seemed like it had come from nowhere. But really, it was there all along—or would've been, if the burden of his weight, his diet, his inactivity, and eventually his diabetes hadn't made him feel so tired for so long.

I wish I could guarantee that everyone reading this will get results like Jason's. Unfortunately, life is never that simple, especially when that life includes a disease like diabetes. What I can promise is that the diet, exercise, and lifestyle-management programs you'll find in the following chapters will help you lose weight, increase your fitness, and improve your health. A lighter, better conditioned, and healthier

# Four Myths about Diabetes

1. **Being overweight causes diabetes.** Obesity is certainly linked to diabetes—globally, obesity and diabetes have increased in tandem—but as you'll see in Chapter 3, not all weight is equally risky. Belly fat has different metabolic effects than fat on other parts of your body, which is why waist size is one of the first measurements I take to assess a patient's health status.

2. **Being thin protects you.** Muscle tissue, as I explain in Chapter 4, is your best defense against diabetes. And, all else being equal, a lean and fit body is almost always a healthy body. But not all thin people are metabolically healthy. Some have more fat (and *much* less muscle) than people classified as overweight or even obese. And in rare cases, people who are both lean and fit develop diabetes. The only way to know for certain is to get your blood tested, especially if you're over 45.

3. **Eating sugar causes diabetes.** As a doctor, I believe we'd all be better off eating fewer foods with added sugar. I can't, however, say that those foods cause diabetes, even though it makes intuitive sense to connect dietary sugar with blood sugar. Diabetes risk escalates with added *food,* not with any one type of food. That said, once you have the disease, or signs that you're at high risk, you absolutely should clean up your diet, starting with highly processed foods that include added sugars.

4. **Once you have diabetes, you have it for life.** This is unfortunately true for type 1 diabetes. With type 2, it's more of a semantic question, a topic I'll tackle in Chapter 15. It's possible to reverse the *symptoms* and regain your health, as you'll see throughout this book, but much harder to determine if underlying issues remain that predispose you to diabetes later in life, especially if you return to doing the things that led you to this point. What I can say without hesitation is that most people in the early stages of the disease can see dramatic improvements, and for some it will be as if they never had it at all.

body is one that's more resistant to just about any disease, especially this one. If you currently have type 2 diabetes, you can lower your dependence on medications, and in some cases stop using them altogether. If you don't yet have it, you can avoid it altogether.

But that's getting ahead of ourselves. Let's take a step back and make sure we understand how you got to this point, what happens if your diabetes goes untreated, and how to ensure your personal journey to recovery becomes a success story, rather than a cautionary tale.

## CHAPTER 2

# What Is Diabetes, and Why Were You at Risk?

IMAGINE THAT YOUR BODY IS a factory. The product you make is energy, and business is booming. You run three 8-hour shifts a day, 7 days a week, 365 days a year. The first two shifts are actively managed by your human staff, while the third shift is fully automated. But even though the lights are out, and no new raw materials are coming in, the machines are still generating that all-important energy.

Our focus here is on the raw materials. Every time you eat a meal or snack, you deliver a new shipment to the factory. Imagine that those materials arrive in trucks to your factory's loading dock. You have a whole staff of workers ready to take the materials off the trucks, and under normal circumstances, it's handled with smooth efficiency.

But then one day there's a problem: It's hard to open the doors of the loading dock. The truck drivers, who in the past simply hit a button on a garage-door opener, now have to hit the button multiple times. When that stops working, they find they need multiple openers for each door. And even when the doors open, they don't always open all the way.

That leaves a pileup of trucks in your loading zone, with the drivers yelling at the guys on the dock to hurry the hell up and get the raw materials off their trucks. The guys on the dock are working as hard as they can, but with partially open doors, it takes much longer to unload each one.

Soon another fleet of trucks arrives at your factory, and now those drivers are upset because they can't pull right up to the loading bays, deliver their materials, and be on their way. Some of the drivers lose patience and abandon their cargo in the parking lot, figuring it's not their problem anymore.

Just when you think it can't get any worse, it does. The management team, confused and exhausted, sees the slowdown as a sign that they should order *more* deliveries, rather than reducing shipments until they get the mess sorted out.

## MEET THE TEAM

A lot of you can guess the names of the players here. The trucks represent your bloodstream, which transports digested nutrients from your most recent meal: carbohydrates (in the form of a sugar called glucose), fat, and protein. The loading bays are your cells. The garage-door openers represent insulin, a hormone that directs nutrients into cells after a meal.

All of your cells use glucose as an energy source, and many of them don't need insulin to tell them what to use or how to use it. Your brain and nervous system, for example, are completely dependent on glucose in most circumstances. (I'll explain some of the nuances and exceptions in later chapters.) Since they use 20 percent of your body's total energy, they soak up a *lot* of that sugar from your blood, without help or hindrance from insulin. But what they can't do is store any significant amount of it. They need your bloodstream to send in a steady supply.

That brings us back to the trucks and garage doors. Your liver, fat cells, and muscles can store glucose. Fat cells either use it for energy or convert it to fat. The liver and muscles convert it to a chemical called glycogen and hoard it for future use. That's one crucial way your brain gets its sugar when there isn't a fresh supply flowing in from your latest meal: Your liver changes glycogen back into glucose, and your brain uses it for energy. But your muscles need insulin—the garage-door opener—for glucose to enter those cells. Your liver needs insulin to turn glucose into glycogen. And your fat cells need insulin to pull both glucose and fat from your bloodstream.

Insulin comes from your pancreas. In type 1 diabetes, as mentioned in Chapter 1, your pancreas either doesn't make the hormone at all, or doesn't make enough. Children with diabetes used to die within months of the symptoms emerging. With the development of purified insulin (originally taken from cattle) in 1921, it ceased to be a death sentence. It was one of the great medical breakthroughs of the 20th century.

In type 2, conversely, the problem isn't a lack of insulin. Not at first, anyway. The cells become insensitive to it. So the pancreas cranks out more. More insulin is not better, for all the reasons that more of anything in a tightly regulated system tends to make things worse. One key hazard: Insulin's role as a gatekeeper works on multiple levels. It directs glucose into liver and muscle cells, fat into fat cells, and protein into muscles. It also keeps glycogen, fat, and protein from *leaving* those cells. Another key responsibility is to temporarily prevent the liver from making glucose out of other nutrients and releasing it into the bloodstream.

In healthy people, the multilevel functions of insulin play nicely with each other. Nutrients flow into cells in the first few hours after a meal. Then, when your body needs nutrients for energy in between meals, they flow right back out. Easy come, easy go. Insensitivity to insulin, followed by an increase in production, throws the whole thing off. It's harder for nutrients to get into cells, but it's also harder to prevent the flow of glucose and fats out of cells, and into your blood, when they aren't needed. The upshot is way too much sugar and fat in circulation.

## WHY YOU?

You have no control over some of the risk factors for diabetes. For example, if a first-degree relative—a parent or sibling—has type 2 diabetes, your risk is several times that of someone with no immediate family history. If you had gestational diabetes during a pregnancy, there's a higher risk later in life. And if you or your ancestors came from Africa, Asia, or Latin America, you have a much greater than average chance of developing diabetes. (Interestingly, it's not the same for all Latinos in the United States. Diabetes rates are highest for Mexican Americans and lowest for Cuban Americans.)

People of European descent, like me, have the lowest risk, possibly because our ancestors invented what's called the Western Diet, with all its highly processed grains and oils. We've thus had the most time to get used to it. Logically, the highest risk would fall on those whose gene pool hears "would you like fries with that?" for the first time.

Whatever your initial risk factors may be, the chance of becoming diabetic increases with your age and weight. (Smoking cigarettes is also linked to diabetes, among many other chronic and deadly diseases. If you smoke, please get whatever help you need to quit.) With age, you naturally tend to slow down. Slowing down means less exercise. Less exercise means smaller and weaker muscles. Those muscles have less active *mitochondria,* which are the parts of cells that generate energy. That makes them less capable of using glucose. Researchers at Yale found that even healthy seniors have 40 percent less mitochondrial activity. Since your muscles typically dispose of 65 percent of the glucose that enters your bloodstream—using it for energy or converting it to glycogen for storage—losing that function is a pretty big deal.

Then there's weight. I'm not here to scold you about the pounds you've put on over the years. Almost every adult with obesity whom I've seen in my practice has tried multiple times to lose weight. I'll discuss this in detail in the next chapter, but for now I'll just say that increasing body weight is strongly linked to diabetes risk, and that the reverse is also true—losing it with diet and exercise has been shown over and over to improve glucose tolerance and insulin sensitivity.

## HOW I KNOW IF YOU HAVE IT

When a patient comes to my office for the first time, I'll automatically check his height and weight and calculate his body mass index, better known as BMI. If you don't know what yours is off the top of your head, take a moment right now to either search for an online calculator, or run the numbers yourself.

1. Multiply your weight in pounds by 0.45.

2. Multiply your height in inches by 0.025, using an online calculator.

3. Calculate the square of step 2 (that is, multiply the number by itself).

4. Divide step 1 by step 3.

As you can see in this chart, each ascending BMI classification is associated with a higher diabetes risk.

| CATEGORY | BMI RANGE | WEIGHT OF A 5'10" MALE (IN POUNDS) | WEIGHT OF A 5'4" FEMALE (IN POUNDS) | ELEVATED DIABETES RISK* |
|---|---|---|---|---|
| Overweight | 25–29.9 | 174–208 | 146–174 | 50% |
| Class I Obesity | 30–34.9 | 209–243 | 175–203 | 150% |
| Class II Obesity | 35–39.9 | 244–278 | 204–232 | 260% |
| Class III Obesity | 40+ | 279+ | 233+ | 410% |

*Compared to those with a BMI in the "ideal" range between 18 and 24.9

I should add here that body mass, by itself, doesn't *cause* diabetes. With a BMI of 28, I'd be in trouble if it did, along with millions of my fellow athletes and serious lifters. BMI is a blunt instrument for judging a patient's health risks. It doesn't distinguish muscle from fat, or take into account how the weight is distributed. Nor does it tell you anything about the patient's diet, exercise, or lifestyle.

That's why I also measure a patient's waistline. It's something you can easily do at home with a cloth measuring tape. Measure right above your hip bones, not around the belly button, which will move as you gain or lose weight. The hip bones are always in the same place, so they give you a more accurate way to keep track over time. The best guideline we have suggests that a waist circumference of 35 inches or more is dangerous for a woman. For a man it's 40 inches or more.

Again, we're just talking about a screening tool to look at potential risk. As with BMI, it doesn't tell the whole story. Some people are born to be thick in the middle, and lots of them are strong, fit, and healthy. There's actually one more screening tool for people who fit that description: waist-to-height ratio (WHtR). It's not one that I use in my office, but some research suggests it's more reliable than BMI or waist circumference for predicting diabetes risk, especially for men. And you can't beat it for simplicity; just divide your waist size in inches by your height in inches.

## WAIST-TO-HEIGHT RATIO (WAIST DIVIDED BY HEIGHT)

| MEN | WOMEN |
|---|---|
| Less than 43%: underweight | Less than 42%: underweight |
| 43%–52%: ideal range | 42%–48%: ideal range |
| 53%–62%: overweight | 49%–57%: overweight |
| 63% or greater: obese | 58% or greater: obese |

At this point I also have a sense of the patient's family and medical history, based on those annoying forms we all have to fill out. (I don't like them any more than you do when I have to slog through them as a patient. But as a doctor, they give me crucial information.) If a patient is overweight on both physical measurements—BMI and waist size—and has additional risk factors, I'm going to ask her to get a fasting plasma glucose test. After 8 or more hours without food, her blood sugar should be under 100 milligrams per deciliter, as you can see in the following chart.

## DIAGNOSTIC TESTS FOR DIABETES

| TEST | NORMAL RANGE | PREDIABETIC | DIABETIC |
|---|---|---|---|
| Fasting blood sugar (mg/dl*) | Less than 100 | 100–125 | 126 or higher |
| Random blood sugar (mg/dl) | Less than 200 | | 200 or higher |
| Hemoglobin A1C | 4%–5.6% | 5.7%–6.4% | 6.5% or higher |
| Oral glucose tolerance (mg/dl) | Less than 140 | 140–199 | 200 or higher |

*mg/dl = milligrams per deciliter of blood

I might also do a random blood sugar test in my office. For that, I can take a drop of blood with a finger stick and measure it with a glucometer. But that's usually reserved for patients like Jason, who, as I described in Chapter 1, gave me good reasons not to put off his diagnosis. I needed that information immediately.

Another valuable test measures hemoglobin A1C, which gives us an average of your blood sugar levels over the past 3 months. Like the random blood sugar test, I can send a patient off for this one without requiring him to fast.

Finally, there's the oral glucose tolerance test. You'd come into the lab after an 8- to 12-hour fast, where they'd measure your blood sugar, give you a glucose drink, and then check your blood sugar 2 hours later. It's most commonly used for pregnant women at risk of gestational diabetes, but it's one I rarely order for my patients because of the time required. I can almost always get the information I need from the other tests.

What I learn from these tests will help me decide on a treatment plan, which may or may not involve medicine. If you're overweight by any of these measures, and if

## JUST A SPOONFUL OF SUGAR...

**... is all a human body is supposed to have in circulation. Here's what happens when you have more than that.**

A healthy body runs throughout the day on a 60-40 mix of fat and glucose. But as you just read, your brain depends entirely on glucose under normal circumstances; fat isn't allowed to cross the blood-brain barrier. So it makes sense that your body would keep a lot of sugar around, since it's the easiest source of energy. And yet it doesn't. A nondiabetic adult who weighs 165 pounds will wake up in the morning with just 5 grams of sugar in his or her bloodstream—a little more than a teaspoon, which is 4.2 grams. Of course that level will rise after meals, but the body's goal is to bring it back down as quickly and efficiently as possible.

*(continued on page 18)*

# Beyond 1 and 2: Four More Types of Diabetes

Most people with diabetes have type 2, and most of us, with or without the disease, know about type 1, in which the pancreas fails to make enough insulin to keep the body alive. But there are actually several others.

## Gestational

Pregnancy mimics obesity in that you gain a lot of weight in your midsection. That by itself causes some insulin resistance, especially in the final weeks. Whether it rises to the level of diabetes depends in part on your insulin sensitivity before you got pregnant. Some women diagnosed early in the pregnancy probably had diabetes or prediabetes before conception, but weren't aware of it.

The biggest risk factors are similar to those for type 2 diabetes, starting with being overweight and inactive before getting pregnant. Women of African, Asian, Native American, or Latin American descent are also at higher risk, as are those who had gestational diabetes with an earlier pregnancy, or who gave birth to a baby who weighed more than 9 pounds.

Gestational diabetes usually goes away when you give birth, but as I noted earlier, it leaves you at higher risk for type 2 diabetes later in life.

## Monogenic

Type 1 and type 2 diabetes are *polygenic,* meaning they're caused by a variety of genes, in combination with lifestyle factors such as obesity in type 2. But a small percentage of cases are *monogenic,* meaning the disease comes from a single gene, which can either be inherited or arise from a spontaneous mutation.

There are two main types.

- *Maturity-onset diabetes of the young (MODY)* may look like type 1 if it develops in childhood, or like type 2 if it's diagnosed later in life. In the latter situation, if there's no family history, the biggest "tell" is that you aren't overweight or you don't have any other obvious risk factors. Your doctor won't know until she orders a genetic test.

- *Neonatal diabetes mellitus (NDM)* develops in infancy—earlier than type 1 usually occurs—and is extremely rare. It can be either permanent or transient. In transient cases, the child grows out of it, but may see it return years later.

## Slow-Onset Type 1 (Type 1.5)

Also known as latent autoimmune diabetes in adults (LADA), it results in high blood sugar, typical of type 2. But it's not because of insulin resistance. Antibodies attack the insulin-producing beta cells of the pancreas, less insulin is produced, and blood glucose rises. As with MODY, the first clue is often the fact that you don't fit the usual profile for type 2. You may be lean and fit, or have normal blood pressure, cholesterol, and triglycerides.

## Pancreatogenic (Type 3c)

Diseases that attack your pancreas—including chronic pancreatitis, cystic fibrosis, and cancer—can damage the organ and leave it incapable of generating enough insulin to control your blood glucose. When diabetes can be linked to one of those conditions, it's classified as type 3c, and is usually preceded by gastrointestinal distress, especially when digesting fat. We know less about pancreatogenic diabetes than any other classification.

you have prediabetes or diabetes, losing weight will be an important part of the plan. How and why are the subjects of the next chapter.

You also know that excess glucose can be converted to glycogen and stored, mostly in the liver and muscles. But even that is a relatively small reserve. An average-size adult might store about 500 grams of glycogen in her muscles and another 100 grams in her liver. If her body used only that stored carbohydrate for energy (it wouldn't, but play along with me here), it might be enough energy to get through a single day. Meanwhile, she probably has at least 30 times that much fat in reserve, providing a month's worth of energy.

One reason you don't hold more carbohydrate is because it's a wet, sloppy mess. Each gram of glycogen in your muscles brings with it 3 grams of water. If you held as much carbohydrate as fat, you'd weigh a *lot* more than you do now. That's why you lose weight so quickly when you switch to a diet that's significantly lower in carbohydrates. Your body stores less glycogen, and subsequently has no need for all the water that supported it.

As for the glucose in your bloodstream, your body works really, really hard to keep it tightly constrained. When it fails, that excess blood sugar does horrible things to virtually every part of your anatomy. At the top of the list:

**Nerve damage (neuropathy).** You may notice a tingling in your fingers or toes, followed by numbness. Imagine how hard it would be to do simple tasks, like filling out a form or writing a check, with numb fingers. Or how hard it would be to walk, much less run, with feet and toes that don't give you the sensory feedback you're accustomed to, or that simply hurt when you put weight on them. Worst-case scenario: You develop sores on your feet that you can't even feel. Those sores, left unchecked, can lead to amputation.

**Cardiovascular disease.** It's not just excess glucose that causes problems. Excess fat is dangerous as well. Insulin resistance leaves you with elevated levels of triglycerides (a type of fat) and a protein called ApoB, which helps form LDL particles. The particles eventually get stuck to the walls of your blood vessels, which makes you several times more likely to have a heart attack or stroke.

**Eye damage (retinopathy).** High blood pressure and high blood lipids put the squeeze on all parts of your circulatory system. It's often seen in the eyes, which have some of the tiniest blood vessels. It can result in blindness, cataracts, or glaucoma.

**Kidney damage (nephropathy).** Your body has a number of systems to clear waste. You can't feel your liver or lymphatic system at work, and you probably don't think much about your lungs, unless you struggle to breathe. But your kidneys force you to pay attention since their efforts send you to the bathroom several times a day. Excessive urination can be one of the warning signs of diabetes, as it was with my patient Jason. You pee more because your kidneys are working so hard to clear that excess glucose from your blood. At the same time, excess lipids can harm the kidneys' intricate network of blood vessels. That can leave you with permanent damage, requiring dialysis and eventually a transplant—*if* you can find a compatible donor.

## CHAPTER 3

# The Benefits of Weight Loss

**I WAS A HEAVYWEIGHT WRESTLER** in college. Because I was nowhere near the upper limit in my weight class, the more mass I could build, the harder it would be to take me down and win the match. But not all weight was equally useful. A few more pounds of lean mass—muscle, bone, and everything else that isn't fat—could translate to significantly more strength without any negative consequences; it wouldn't make me slower or disrupt my balance. Extra fat, on the other hand, did me no good at all.

Of course we all need some fat. The brain, for example, is about 60 percent fat, once you drain the water. (Brains, like muscles, are about 75 percent $H_2O$.) Fat helps provide structure to our cells and is a crucial source of energy throughout the day. The leanest athletes you see on TV, like gymnasts or sprinters or figure skaters, still have some essential fat on their bodies. They couldn't function without it. But a strange thing happens when you have too much fat: It develops a mind of its own.

# THE BELLY OF THE BEAST

Until the 1980s, most scientists who study the human body believed that fat cells were inert. Like your neighbor's lazy cat, they just sat around waiting to be fed. We now know they do a lot more. Fat tissue is actually an *endocrine system,* which means it generates hormones and also responds to them. It communicates with your brain and even has a role in your immune system. The more fat you have, the more power it assumes over the rest of your body.

In some ways it's actually multiple endocrine systems, releasing and reacting to different hormones in different ways, depending on where the fat is located. There are two major types.

- **Subcutaneous fat** sits between your skin and muscles. You recognize it as love handles, double chins, upper-arm jiggle (aka batwings), and the thigh fat that women's bodies preferentially accumulate (even though very few women would *prefer* to have it there, if given a choice).

- **Ectopic fat** develops when your subcutaneous cells run out of room, or for various reasons can't take in any new fat from your blood. The excess fat gathers in places it's not supposed to be, including your internal organs (visceral fat), your liver (fatty liver), and your muscle cells (intramuscular fat).

Leptin, an appetite-regulating hormone, is generated primarily in subcutaneous fat. It operates on what we call a negative feedback loop—more of one thing causes less of something else. In this case, more leptin means less hunger and a lower appetite. The more fat you have, the more leptin those cells produce, and the less hunger you should experience. The converse is also true: When you get leaner, you generate less leptin and experience more hunger. It makes sense if you think of leptin as a hormone that evolved to regulate your weight by keeping you from storing too little or too much fat.

Unfortunately, leptin is no match for our modern food chain, which makes it too easy to eat when we aren't hungry. Excess food creates excess fat. Excess fat creates excess leptin. But instead of that leptin shutting down your appetite, your body becomes less responsive to it. It's similar to the way your muscle and fat cells become insensitive to insulin.

Things get even worse when ectopic fat begins to accumulate. That's because, unlike subcutaneous fat, it has direct access to vital organs. Hormones and fatty acids from visceral fat flow straight into the liver, where they disrupt your metabolism and contribute to both obesity and insulin resistance, and by extension to diabetes and cardiovascular disease.

Then there's intramuscular fat, something we all have in small amounts. For endurance athletes, especially females, it's an important energy source since it sits right next to the muscle fibers that need it. But that fat stops being useful when you develop type 2 diabetes. You accumulate it faster but lose your ability to burn it during exercise.

It's an insidious cycle: Ectopic fat releases chemicals that either lead to or exacerbate insulin resistance. Insulin resistance makes your muscles less responsive to exercise. Muscles that can't respond to exercise accumulate intramuscular fat, which the muscles can't burn as efficiently as they should. Then the presence of that intramuscular fat makes the muscles even more dysfunctional, which means you get less benefit from exercise, which makes everything worse.

I tell you all this for a very important reason: Losing any amount of weight—a little, a lot, or anything in between—improves your health in measurable, substantial, and sometimes dramatic ways.

## A LITTLE OFF THE MIDDLE

Everyone seems to agree that losing 5 to 10 percent of your weight is beneficial. Insulin sensitivity improves; blood sugar, blood pressure, and triglycerides decline; HDL cholesterol (the beneficial kind) typically rises. All good news so far, right? The disconnect occurs when official organizations like the US Centers for Disease Control and Prevention describe this degree of weight loss as "modest." It's like there's a value attached to it. If we're talking about a modest house or a modest car or a modest lifestyle, we're saying it's inexpensive and easily acquired. Many of my patients would disagree.

For a 160-pound woman, a "modest" reduction of 5 to 10 percent would be 8 to 16 pounds. For a man weighing in at 220, it's 11 to 22 pounds. Most who try to lose weight will tell you there's nothing easy about it. But as their doctor, I know it's worth the effort.

Consider the results of the Look AHEAD (Action for Health in Diabetes) study. It involved more than 5,000 middle-aged adults with diabetes, about 60 percent of them women. Their average starting weight was 220 pounds. Half of them partici-

## SHOULD YOU CONSIDER WEIGHT-LOSS SURGERY?

Bariatric surgery seems like an odd topic for a book promising a "natural" approach. But as I said in the Introduction, there's nothing natural about any aspect of modern life that increases our weight and compromises our health. Surgery, while expensive and not always covered by insurance, has an extraordinarily high success rate for those with diabetes. It's so successful, in fact, that while I was working on these opening chapters, the journal *Diabetes Care* published a joint statement recommending surgery as a treatment option. The authors are highly credentialed experts from across the globe, backed by dozens of medical organizations.

The best candidates, they say, are those with a BMI of 35 or above and persistent high blood sugar despite taking measures to reduce it. They add that surgery should also be considered an option for patients with a BMI of 30 to 34.9. (For Asians, the BMI cutoffs are 2.5 points lower.)

Roux-en-Y gastric bypass, which reroutes your intestines and reduces your

pated in an intensive weight-loss program, while the other half got less personalized guidance—group classes along with the usual "eat less, move more" advice.

After 1 year, 65 percent of the volunteers in the intensive group dropped at least 5 percent of their initial weight, achieving the minimum for "modest" weight loss. After 4 years, 46 percent still weighed at least 5 percent less. And after 8 years, interestingly, that number had grown to 50 percent.

Fifty percent is an impressive result over that many years. Also impressive: Among the volunteers in the *other* group, the ones who mostly just got conventional advice, 36 percent had lost at least 5 percent when the study ended.

There wouldn't be any point in mentioning all this unless "modest" weight loss

stomach to the size of an egg, is the best-known weight-loss surgery and has the highest success rate for those with diabetes. Patients typically see their blood sugar and insulin levels return to normal within days, way before they lose any serious amount of weight. Even doctors aren't exactly sure why this happens so suddenly. Eating a lot less food is obviously part of it, along with the fact that you absorb fewer nutrients from your teeny-tiny meals. Altering the anatomy of your digestive system is another factor. Those changes in turn affect hormones and gut bacteria. Another line of thought suggests that the sudden drop in calories reduces fat in the liver and pancreas, improving the function of both organs.

But it's important to know that these changes aren't always permanent. Up to half of the patients whose diabetes was resolved eventually see it return. That's why it's crucial that you continue to do everything I talk about in this book—exercise, make good food choices, monitor and manage your weight carefully, and make sure you get a good night's sleep.

delivers meaningful benefits, which it most certainly does. The researchers found significant reductions in blood sugar, hemoglobin A1C, blood pressure, and triglycerides, and a nice increase in HDL cholesterol. The more weight the participants lost, the more they improved in all those measures.

That's the good news. Unfortunately, 5 percent does seem to be the cutoff between significant and nonsignificant improvements. In most studies that last a year or more, the average loss is less than 5 percent of the volunteers' starting weight, and the benefits fall below the standard of statistical significance. But that doesn't mean small changes don't matter. They do.

## Four Myths about Weight Loss

1. **All weight-loss efforts are doomed to fail.** If you read a lot about health and nutrition, you've probably come across this statement: "Ninety-five percent of all diets fail." I assume that number comes from somewhere. But it doesn't reflect the latest research. In the Look AHEAD study I described earlier, 50 percent of those in the intensive-intervention group kept a meaningful amount of weight off for 8 years, as did 36 percent of those who got much less help. This was a major study with more than 5,000 volunteers. Nor does the 95 percent statistic reflect my experience. I have patients who lost weight in my first year of practice and have kept it off ever since.

2. **Rapid weight loss leads to rapid weight regain, leaving you worse off than before.** Crash diets have a deservedly bad reputation, especially if they're marketed with words like "detox" or "cleanse." Everything about those diets is stupid and fraudulent. Much of the lost weight is from muscle tissue, and losing muscle does indeed predispose you to regain everything you lost, and then some. Same with those crazy, sadistic regimens you see on *The Biggest Loser*. But in clinical studies, the opposite is actually true. The

# SMALL CHANGES, BIG RESULTS

I could come up with a long list of reasons why I can't stand the way we talk about weight loss. I already mentioned my least favorite: "Eat less, move more." Yes, in general, it's exactly what most of us need to do. But without actual guidance on *how* to modify your diet and *how* to work more physical activity into your life, it's useless. It allows the dispenser of this advice (usually someone for whom weight control is relatively easy) to feel good about himself, while it makes the recipient of the advice feel worse.

more weight subjects lose, and the faster they lose it, the less they weigh by the end of the follow-up period. The truth is that there's no right or wrong pace. Losing weight quickly doesn't mean you're any more likely to regain it.

3. **A diet has to be extreme to work.** I'm agnostic when it comes to diets. I have a preference for the Mediterranean diet (or at least my own interpretation of it). I'll explain why in Chapter 10. But if one of my patients wants to try an extreme low-fat or low-carb or paleo or vegan or raw-food diet, I'm going to help her set up the healthiest possible version of that diet. Decades of research have shown that no diet is objectively better than any other. Adherence matters more than anything else, and the only way to stick to a diet over the long term is to start with one that you like.

4. **Weight loss is a character issue, reflecting your willpower and commitment.** Hunger isn't a test of your personal integrity. It's a biological signal telling you to eat something. You're *supposed* to pay attention to it. Ignoring it is unnatural; very few of us can do it for long. I'll take a closer look at the biology and physiology of hunger in Chapter 6. For now I'll just say this: Your goal isn't to ignore hunger. It's to avoid it altogether.

Then there's the way my fellow doctors use BMI to label two-thirds of Americans as overweight or obese; as I noted, *I'm* overweight by that standard, as are many adults who are both strong and fit. Meanwhile, lots of people get a clean bill of health from their doctors because their BMI is in the "ideal" range, or shows that they're only moderately overweight, when in fact they have a lot of ectopic fat and are at high risk for everything we've talked about in this book.

But perhaps the most deflating conversations are the ones that start like this: "My goal is to lose XXX pounds." The moment you put such a specific number on your aspirations, you handicap yourself. Anything short of that number represents failure. And when it comes to weight loss, there's really no such thing as failure. As long as you're trying, you're succeeding.

Think of it this way.

- Focusing on your weight automatically shifts your attitude about food. You think before you eat. You make plans. You develop strategies.

- When you focus on what you're eating, and how you're eating it, you make better choices.

- Making better choices usually means eating less food, or at least choosing foods with less added sugar and fat.

Even if all those adjustments don't produce weight loss, they do help you with weight *control*. The average American adult gains a pound or two a year. If you have diabetes and obesity, in a typical year you probably put on more than that. *Not gaining more weight* is a crucial step toward improving your health. Maintaining your current weight for 2 or 3 years is the equivalent of losing all the weight you would have gained. And there's nothing to prevent you from losing weight in the future.

I'll go into much more detail about nutrition and weight loss in Part Two. But before we get into all that, the next two chapters will look at exercise and sleep, both of which are absolutely essential to anyone who wants to beat diabetes.

## CHAPTER 4

# The Magic of Exercise

**I LOVE TO WORK OUT.** I love to push myself as hard as I can for as long as I can. Furthermore, I love to compete against other guys who push themselves as hard as I do. That's why I wrestled and played football in college, and why I competed in bodybuilding when I was 30. I even trained for and completed a triathlon, despite knowing I'd be mediocre at best. I thought of it as a competition against myself, to see if I could build endurance in running, swimming, and cycling with my strength-trained body while still lifting heavy weights. It was every bit as hard as it sounds, and I loved (almost) every minute of it.

But for some of my patients, the thought of doing *any* exercise is as intimidating as climbing a mountain or jumping out of an airplane might be for me. That may describe you as well. If so, I can guess how you respond to guidelines like the following, which the American Diabetes Association promotes as the standard for adults with diabetes.

- "Moderate to vigorous aerobic exercise" for at least 150 minutes a week

- "Moderate to vigorous resistance training" at least 2 or 3 days a week

- "Milder forms of physical activity"—like tai chi and yoga—"have shown mixed results"

- "Flexibility training" is okay, "but should not be undertaken in place of other recommended types of physical activity"

Is that encouraging to you? Do you feel inspired to hop up from the couch and go do what some committee of people in lab coats says you should? Don't get me wrong: I'd love it if all my patients, and everyone reading this book, exercised at least 30 minutes a day. I'm 100 percent in favor of strength training several days a week. Furthermore, I'm familiar with the research that underpins the guidelines, so I understand how they settled on these numbers. But they do nothing to help people get from where they are to where they could be, and that bothers the hell out of me.

Exercise is as potent as anything I can recommend or prescribe. It prevents more diseases, reverses more conditions, adds more years to life, and does more to improve the quality of that life. But I can't just write my exercise prescription on a piece of paper and send you to the pharmacy for a bottle of fitness. And to be honest, even if I could, I wouldn't want to. Stick with me for a few minutes, and I'll explain why.

## WHAT IS EXERCISE?

I assume this book's readers are as diverse as the patients I see in my practice. Some of you have a regular fitness routine, but many more are struggling to get started. You know you're *supposed* to exercise—you can't turn on the TV, open a magazine, or go out in public without being reminded of it. But you don't know where to begin, and your previous attempts didn't leave you with high hopes that you ever will.

If that applies to you, let's try an experiment. I want you to put down this book and stand up.

Done?

Great. Now, sit down again.

You know what just happened? You exercised! You got up from the chair, using muscles in your hips and thighs—the biggest, strongest, and most metabolically active skeletal muscles you have—and then you sat down again, engaging those same muscles, along with others in your torso and feet to keep your body balanced and stabilized.

Let's try another experiment.

Set the book down again. Stand up again. Now walk across the room and back before you return to your chair. You exercised again, but this time you did more.

That's really all there is to it. You get up. You move. Every minute you spend on your feet, supporting your own weight while moving around, forces your body to make countless adjustments. Your nervous system activates muscles. Glucose and fat in your bloodstream provide energy to those muscles, which has two crucial benefits: You clear sugar and lipids from your blood, and you burn more calories. Prolonged exercise, especially at a relatively vigorous pace (it *feels* like exercise, in other words), does even more: It temporarily elevates your metabolism and keeps it elevated for an hour or two after you finish. A higher metabolic rate speeds up everything. Your heart beats a little faster. Your lungs take in more oxygen. More nutrients flow into and out of your blood, your muscles, and your fat cells. Your cells become more sensitive to insulin because they need those nutrients that insulin is in charge of clearing from your blood.

Here's how powerful exercise is: Physical activity reduces the risk of developing type 2 diabetes by 50 to 80 percent.

Which is great to know if you don't yet have diabetes. With regular exercise and some measure of dietary restraint (that is, you don't approach each meal like it's potentially your last), you can probably avoid it altogether, no matter how many risk factors you were born with.

But even for those who have diabetes, there's also some pretty good news. In a study published in *Diabetes Care* in 2016, an Australian research team showed that a minimal amount of exercise significantly reduced post-meal glucose, insulin, and triglyceride levels. The researchers had their volunteers get up from their chairs every 30 minutes and either walk around for 3 minutes or do a 3-minute routine of simple lower-body exercises, like half squats and calf raises. The volunteers, all of whom had type 2 diabetes, may or may not resemble you. The average age was 62; they were inactive and spent at least 5 hours a day sitting, and they were all considered overweight or obese, according to BMI. If they can get all those improvements with just 24 nonconsecutive minutes of exercise, imagine what you could do with a little more time and effort.

## WHY YOU SHOULD GO LONG

When doctors and scientists talk about exercise, they usually divide it into two categories: aerobic training, which most of us refer to as cardio; and strength or resistance training, often described simply as lifting. The terminology suggests there's a clear line between the two, but in real life the line is pretty blurry, if it exists at all.

Let's say you join a gym, with the goal of doing my basic program, shown in Chapter 12. You go from doing nothing to working out for 30 to 45 minutes three times a week. Technically, it's *strength* training, and you should indeed get stronger. But you'll almost certainly improve your aerobic fitness as well. You'll notice how much easier it is to move around and handle life's most mundane tasks, which you may currently avoid because they leave you out of breath. That's the combined result of improved strength—each step takes a little less effort—and better endurance. You'll also move faster, thanks to improved muscle strength and power. And for good measure, you'll probably end up with better balance and flexibility. All from doing a type of exercise that's marketed to people who want stronger, sexier muscles.

But for all the benefits of strength training—including a big one that I haven't yet described—the best evidence we have suggests that aerobic exercise is the most reliable way to defeat diabetes.

I already mentioned that your muscles hold a few hundred grams of glycogen, which they make from glucose. Muscle glycogen can only be used to power muscle activity. Aerobic exercise, with its repetitive use of your body's biggest muscles, drains a lot of glycogen, which your muscles quickly replace with glucose from the bloodstream.

That's why I encourage my inactive patients to start with walking. It doesn't matter how far you walk at first, or how fast. As long as it's more than you were doing before, it's great. A little more? Even better. Can you go a bit faster? Better still. Can you mix up your speeds, so you alternate between your normal walking speed and a faster pace, one that starts to feel like exercise? Awesome. And you can make it even more beneficial by finding a route that includes some hills. The change in elevation will add a mild strength-boosting and muscle-developing effect, on top of all the other benefits.

As a reward for doing more, you reverse just about every condition linked to diabetes. You will:

- Lower your blood sugar, A1C, and triglycerides

- Improve insulin sensitivity

- Improve cardiovascular health (lower your blood pressure and resting heart rate, increase your capillary networks)

- Decrease body fat

- Decrease visceral fat

- Lower your risk of both heart disease and overall mortality

Not bad for something you learned to do when you were still in diapers!

## WHY YOU SHOULD GET STRONG

*Muscle quality* is a measure of your strength relative to the size of your muscles. It's associated not only with better physical performance, but also with a lower risk of diabetes and a longer life. Adults with diabetes typically have lower muscle quality than those without the disease. They have larger muscles, on average, but less strength.

# A Few Words of Caution

When I encourage a patient to start a fitness program, we both know she has her doctor's approval. But when I talk about exercise with readers like you, it's with the understanding that you'll discuss it with your own doctor, especially if you're just starting out.

Hypoglycemia is a concern if you're currently taking insulin for type 1 or type 2 diabetes. Exercise disrupts the delicate balance of food and medicine, and it can potentially leave you with too little glucose in your blood. You're at risk at two different times: during and immediately after exercise; and up to 11 hours later, when your muscles are still working to replenish glycogen. So before you begin any fitness program, you need to consult with your doctor on a recalibration strategy.

Cardiovascular disease is another big risk factor. Exercise increases both your heart rate and the amount of blood your heart pumps with each beat. That blood, carrying oxygen and nutrients, has to reach every nook and cranny in your circulatory system. Then it has to carry carbon dioxide and other waste products back to your heart. Any chinks in your circulatory system—like blocked blood vessels or weak arterial walls—could have disastrous consequences. And yet, you need exercise; it's the only way to strengthen your heart and improve your overall health. Research and practice show it's both safe and effective. You just need to make sure your doctor is aware of and approves your program.

You also have to take your joints and extremities into consideration. Even walking puts added pressure on your feet, ankles, knees, hips, and lower back. (Jogging puts even more stress on them.) If you have problems with your feet related to diabetes, or knee pain related to your weight or previous injuries, a doctor or physical therapist can help you modify your fitness program to avoid making those things worse.

In Chapter 3 I talked about the dangers of storing fat in places where it shouldn't be. Intramuscular fat is highly correlated with lower muscle quality, which isn't at all surprising. It doesn't matter which came first—if lower quality allowed more intramuscular fat to accumulate, or if the fat caused a drop in strength. The problem is the same: Your muscles don't work as well as they should.

With weaker, fattier muscles, your body can do less, and you get less benefit from what you do. Simple chores and light exercise are harder, take longer, and burn fewer calories. You use less glycogen from your muscles, which means your muscles subsequently pull less glucose from your blood.

Strength training reverses all these negative trends. Strength and muscle quality increase. Physical performance improves. You move faster, go farther, and burn more calories in the process. You also make your muscles a little bigger. I'm sure that's a scary thought for some of you, but it shouldn't be. For one thing, you have to do a *lot* of lifting to build enough muscle for anyone to notice. For another, the new muscle you build is unlikely to increase your weight. Any exercise program will help you lose fat, and the worst outcome of a strength-training program is that you break even, gaining muscle and losing fat in roughly equal amounts. Even then, you end up with a leaner body, since muscle tissue is more compact.

Now, you may have noticed that I've been talking about cardio and strength training in binary terms, which I said earlier I don't really like to do. But if I'm going to talk about specific benefits, I have to divide things up the way researchers do in high-quality studies. So if they study aerobic exercise, they have their volunteers walk or run on treadmills, or pedal stationary bikes. If it's a strength-training study, the subjects typically work out on machines, which is also what they use to measure strength before and after. It's not how I would set up workout programs for my patients, unless that's what they tell me they want to do. But it's a valuable and honest way to do scientific research because it ensures everyone in the study is doing the same things in the same way. (If you've spent much time in health clubs, you know that's totally *not* the norm.)

Which brings me to my last big point.

## "ALL OF THE ABOVE" IS SIMPLER THAN IT SOUNDS

If cardio training offers one set of benefits, and strength training offers another, you might assume that some combination of the two would work best. The research says you'd be right. That's why the official recommendation for adults with diabetes is to

## FOUR MYTHS ABOUT EXERCISE

1. **Exercise is a great way to lose weight.** Not long ago, doctors and exercise scientists believed that weight loss was a simple matter of calories-in, calories-out. If you increased the calories going out with exercise, you should lose weight. That's just math. But decades of weight-loss research have shown the opposite: On average, your weight won't change very much. You're doing pretty well if you lose a few pounds over any given period of time with exercise alone.

2. **You can't lose weight with exercise.** This was the knee-jerk reaction to studies showing those modest results. But it's really more complicated than that. A landmark 2008 study in the *International Journal of Obesity* highlighted the problem with focusing on "average" weight loss. The study included 35 sedentary men and women with obesity, all of whom did a fairly high volume of exercise for 12 weeks. Average weight loss was 8 pounds, which isn't bad. But the individual range was enormous: One person lost 32 pounds, while another gained 4. You could be a super-responder to exercise, a non-responder, or anything in between. There's only one way to find out.

3. **Exercise just makes you hungrier.** It might or it might not. Logically, though, an ambitious fitness routine *should* make you hungrier. Your body isn't stupid. If your workouts drain energy from your muscles and fat cells, *of course* your body will want more food to replace it. It's a feature, not a

do both, as I mentioned: 150 minutes a week of cardio, plus two or three strength workouts. But is that really the best approach?

In theory, maybe. In practice, no. I've never had a patient who jumped right into a routine like that, and very few who eventually managed to build up to it. Even people without obesity or diabetes rarely get that much exercise. For that matter,

bug. But that doesn't mean the food you take in has to make you fatter. It takes calories to process calories, so when you eat more, you also burn more during digestion—especially when you're eating higher-protein meals, as I'll discuss in detail in Part Two. It's certainly easy to overdo the "eat more" part of the equation; you don't need me to tell you that. I just want to reassure you there's no reason to fear post-workout food.

4. **"[Fill in the blank] is the best workout in the world!" The basic principles of a good workout have been understood for almost as long as humans have exercised.** It starts with *progressive overload*—gradually doing more or lifting more. (Describe it twice in this chapter.) Progress is linear at first. Your strength or endurance increases workout to workout, week to week, month to month. And then you run head-on into the limitations of your schedule, your individual capacity, or the number of times you can do the same thing without getting bored. That's when you need to shake things up with a new plan, or a fresh variation on what you're already doing. Long-time exercisers are fond of saying that the best workout for you is the one you haven't yet tried, which makes sense. But that's very different from deciding your new program is best for *everybody*. It might be the right choice for you, or your coworker, or whoever is endorsing it, *at this particular moment*. But for almost everyone else, it's just one of many options.

healthy, fit people who love to work out almost never conform to the guidelines either. And yet they're still healthy and fit.

It really comes down to this: We all hate being told we *have* to do something. That's equally true of those who look forward to their workouts and those who loathe the very idea of working up a sweat. In that sense, finding the right exercise program is very much like finding the right diet. You have to start with something you enjoy, or at minimum tolerate. If that's walking, or lifting weights, or doing yoga, or pedaling a stationary bike in your basement while catching up on *Dancing with the Stars,* great. We'll call that Step 1 and start there.

**Step 2: *Do a little more.*** Walk a little farther. Pedal a little longer. Do another yoga class. Add some exercises to your weight routine.

**Step 3: *Improve your performance.*** Walk faster. Pedal harder. Sign up for a more challenging yoga class. Focus on lifting heavier weights.

**Step 4: *Shift gears.*** Add some intervals to a cardio routine—go faster than your normal speed for 60 seconds, then a little slower for 60 seconds. Take a non-yoga class at your gym, like spinning, to challenge yourself in a new way. If you're a lifter, cut down the rest periods between sets and exercises, and do some exercises a little faster. (You'll find much more guidance for this and the previous step in Part Three.)

**Step 5: *Add something new.*** Try some calisthenics, or basic resistance exercises with dumbbells or bands, at the beginning or end of your cardio routine. After yoga class, do a circuit of exercises on the weight machines—one set of each, 10 to 12 repetitions, increasing the weight when the final rep starts to feel easy. Lifters can finish a strength workout with 20 minutes on the treadmill or stationary bike.

If you make it to Step 5, you'll probably find you enjoy the adjunct exercises more than you expected. I know it's hard to imagine if you're at Step 1, but it really is fun to challenge yourself in a new way. Importantly, the goal isn't to become good at this new part of your routine, unless you want to. It's to become better at the thing you already like to do. Runners run faster when they're a little stronger, with fewer injuries, while aerobic fitness helps lifters do more lifting.

All that is in addition to what may be the biggest bonus of diversifying your fitness portfolio: You get leaner, partly as a result of doing more exercise, and partly because you've pushed your body to adapt to something new. A body that can do more tends to *look* like a body that can do more.

Now you can see why I wouldn't want to prescribe a pill that makes you fit, even if such a thing were available. The real benefits of exercise begin with the personal satisfaction you get from overcoming inertia, from getting up and moving, from showing gravity your middle finger, from proving to yourself and to anyone who doubted you that diabetes doesn't have the final word.

## CHAPTER 5

# Sleep Your Way to Better Health

**SO FAR I'VE ASKED YOU** to lose weight and start an exercise program, or ramp up the one you're already doing. I tried to explain weight loss and exercise in the least intimidating way possible, but I understand how daunting they will seem to many of you. I get the same reaction every day in my practice.

Now I'm going to ask you to make one more lifestyle adjustment. Fortunately, it's one you can do in your sleep. Because it *is* sleep.

Poor sleep is associated with almost every problem we've discussed in this book: high blood sugar, poor insulin sensitivity, increased weight, increased waist size, obesity, and diabetes. But before we can discuss "poor sleep," and how to improve it, we should look at something more fundamental.

## WHAT IS SLEEP?

It's 11:00 p.m., but of course you don't know that because you conked out a half-hour ago. You're now in slow-wave sleep, the deepest stage. Your heart rate, blood pressure, and body temperature all drop, and your brain uses much less glucose. Growth hormone peaks during slow-wave sleep, which makes sense, since this is the time when your body does its heaviest lifting to rebuild and repair tissues, and that's exactly what growth hormone does. Also increasing is ghrelin, a hormone that stimulates hunger. If you happen to sleepwalk, this is when you'd do it—and, thanks to the rise in ghrelin, people who sleepwalk might also sleep-eat. Your body is hungry, but it doesn't expect you to do anything about it.

After about an hour, you shift out of deep sleep and briefly reach REM sleep, which is when most dreams happen. That's the way it goes for the rest of the night: You alternate between cycles of deep (or deep-ish) sleep, dream-rich REM sleep, and brief moments when you're either awake, or nearly so.

It's almost impossible to overstate how important all these phases are. In addition to the physical restoration that happens during the deepest sleep, we know this is when your brain consolidates and organizes memories. Your brain even rehearses movements—physical memories—during REM sleep. (It cuts off the signaling hormones that would make your body move during these rehearsals. Your eyes are moving like crazy, but your arms, legs, and torso are immobile.)

One more crucial role of sleep: During the day your brain accumulates substances called amyloid proteins. Think of them as metabolic trash. New research suggests that sleep gives your brain the opportunity to send fluid in to flush the garbage out. If you've heard of amyloid proteins, it's because they're associated with Alzheimer's disease. Those who get Alzheimer's are less efficient at clearing them away, and the accumulation could lead to dementia. Now we know from animal research that your body has an overnight cleaning crew that can do its job only when you're sound asleep.

Over the past half-century or so, Americans have curtailed their sleep by an estimated 1.5 to 2 hours per night. During that same time the rates of obesity and diabetes have risen dramatically. That doesn't mean poor sleep *causes* obesity or diabetes, but there's good reason to believe they're connected in a destructive loop. Here's how it works.

**Step 1:** You get less sleep, for whatever reason—shift work, stress and anxiety, or personal choices, like staying up late to watch TV or play computer games.

**Step 2:** Shortened or disrupted sleep throws off key hormones that regulate appetite. Ghrelin, which is supposed to rise during deep sleep, remains low at night but rises during the day. Leptin, the hunger-regulating hormone we discussed in Chapter 3, falls. The combination of higher ghrelin and lower leptin increases your appetite in general, and lack of sleep increases specific cravings for sugar and fat. You also burn fewer calories during the day because of a drop in a key thyroid hormone.

**Step 3:** Cortisol, a stress hormone, rises, along with a group of hormones linked to inflammation. These trigger insulin resistance, even in healthy young people who aren't overweight.

**Step 4:** Eating more, moving less, and struggling to process glucose and other nutrients in your blood lead to weight gain, which not only puts you at higher risk for diabetes, but also makes it harder to get a good night's sleep.

**Step 5:** Worse sleep exacerbates all these hormonal disruptions, making it easier to gain weight and much harder to do anything about it. Your body craves the very foods you're trying to avoid, and when you're chronically exhausted, exercise is the last thing you can motivate yourself to do.

Consistently good sleep does the opposite.

- You'll be less hungry during the day, and less likely to crave the doughnuts and potato chips and greasy cheeseburgers that you know you should avoid.

- You'll be more active in general, and much more likely to stick with your fitness routine.

- You'll have better blood sugar control, with less insulin resistance.

But before I show you how to improve your sleep, I need to explain why it's so hard for someone who's seriously overweight.

# HOW OBESITY PUTS YOU IN A CHOKE HOLD

I screen every single patient who comes into my office for obstructive sleep apnea. It falls under the category of sleep-disordered breathing, which affects an estimated 34 percent of men and 17 percent of women between the ages of 30 and 70. A few signs that you may have it:

- **You snore, choke, or gasp for breath when sleeping.** Not everyone who snores has sleep apnea, but everyone with sleep apnea snores. Most of them snore *hard*. You've heard sleep referred to as sawing logs or cutting *z's*? Sleep apnea makes you sound like you're cutting wood with a chain saw while riding a Harley in a parking garage.

- **You wake up feeling tired.** At the end of four or five normal sleep cycles, you should feel refreshed and ready to handle whatever life throws your way.

- **You're tired throughout the day.** It's not normal to doze off in meetings, no matter how boring they are, or to spend much of the day feeling as if your brain is running at half speed. Nor is it good for your career; all things being equal, a sleep-deprived employee will perform far worse than her well-rested colleagues.

- **You have a big neck.** A neck circumference larger than 17 inches in men and 16 inches in women is a red flag. The bigger the neck, the more tissue there is to potentially cause an obstruction. And that's what sleep apnea is: You've blocked the airway with your own flesh, and without sufficient oxygen, your body goes into panic mode and forces you to wake up.

Lack of oxygen has a number of effects that may seem unrelated to sleep, like waking up with a headache or developing high blood pressure. Several of my male patients with low testosterone saw it rebound to normal levels when they lost weight and resolved their sleep disorders.

Yes, I mentioned weight loss. Again. Losing 5 percent of your body weight can help reduce the problem, especially if your apnea falls into the mild or moderate range.

But I won't try to blow any smoke down your obstructed throat. Research shows that it takes *significant* weight loss to clear up the problem entirely.

Because I can't diagnose sleep apnea in my office, much less classify it on a scale from mild to severe, I often refer my patients to a sleep specialist. If that doctor shares my concern, he'll have the patients spend the night in a sleep clinic, where they'll be observed and evaluated. Trust me, I know how weird it seems to have

## NEED TO LOSE WEIGHT? SLEEP ON IT!

When Sean first came to my practice, he had almost a textbook example of a diabetes-inducing lifestyle. He was 40, with a couple of young kids and a demanding job that required him to get up early in the morning. He was also seriously overweight.

Sean told me he was trying to lose weight, and was ready and willing to implement the diet and fitness plan we put together. But he was always too tired to follow through. Too tired to exercise, too tired to cook healthy meals.

The problem, I soon realized, was his nighttime routine. He'd stay up late watching TV, and he was lucky to get 4 or 5 hours of sleep before he had to wake up to start another exhausting day.

So that's what we focused on. We counted backward from his daily wake-up time and made a rule that the TV had to be off at least 8 hours before then. Without the TV to keep him awake, he found it much easier to fall asleep at a reasonable time, and averaged 2 more hours of sleep each night.

More sleep, and better sleep, made everything else fall into place. He woke up each morning with more energy. He moved more during the day, stuck to his exercise schedule, and cooked meals at night instead of ordering takeout.

And his weight, which he'd struggled with for years, started falling steadily without any changes in our original diet and exercise plan. It was as easy as falling asleep.

strangers watching you sleep. My patients are never comfortable with the idea at first. But it helps to think of it from the point of view of the professionals at the clinic. Do you think there's anything you would do in your sleep that they haven't seen before? Any noises you would make that they haven't heard?

If their observations and measurements confirm that you have sleep apnea, they'll likely have you return for another night, this time using CPAP (continuous positive airway pressure), a machine that pushes air past the constriction and into your lungs. Or, if your apnea is obvious and severe, the doctor may try CPAP midway through that first night in the clinic.

Again, I appreciate how reluctant my patients are to use the machine. It looks like

## Short-Term Benefit, Long-Term Danger

In the past, doctors sometimes recommended a medication like diphenhydramine (Benadryl) to help those with allergies fall asleep and stay asleep. It's an easy and immediate fix, since the pills are cheap and don't require a prescription. They also help knock you out fast. But we now know there's a terrifying side effect: Diphenhydramine is linked to a higher risk of Alzheimer's. The more you take, and the longer you take it, the higher the risk. Animal studies show that it prevents your brain from cleaning out the amyloid proteins that lead to dementia, allowing the plaque to accumulate.

Today we have much safer allergy pills, like loratadine (Claritin). But even with those, you still want to keep your bedroom as clean as possible, including your sheets and blankets. You can also defend your sleep cave against allergenic intruders by changing your clothes before entering, especially if you've worn those clothes outside or around a pet.

And just because nothing in medicine is simple, you should take allergy pills only when absolutely necessary, since they've been linked to weight gain.

a minimalist scuba mask, with one strap around your forehead and another holding the part of the device that covers your nose and forces air into it, and reminds you of the ventilators they use in hospitals for severely injured or terminally ill patients. It takes some convincing to get them to try it. Once they do, it's like they've been transported back in time. They wake up refreshed, with energy and optimism. They're more patient with their spouses and children, more productive at work, more likely to follow through on their commitment to eat better and exercise.

I've had a number of patients who diagnosed themselves with attention deficit disorder and asked me about taking a stimulant like Adderall. But what they really needed was to breathe while asleep. Once they addressed the sleep problem, and didn't wake up tired and brain-fogged every morning, the ADD went away.

## SWEET DREAMS ARE MADE OF THIS

There are many ways to improve your sleep quality short of CPAP, or in conjunction with it. Among them are the following:

### Don't Go into the Light

Each of us has a natural body clock. I tend to be a morning person, but you may be the opposite. Whichever it is, you need to give yourself every chance to fall asleep according to your own circadian rhythms. The last thing you want to do is hit your retinas with direct light before bedtime, especially from an electronic device. Not only does direct light upset your internal clock, electronic entertainment will stimulate your brain in other ways. *That's what it's supposed to do.* No one ever designed a game, or produced a TV show, or created a social-media platform with the goal of helping the audience fall asleep.

A recent Japanese study found that those who got the most nighttime light exposure increased both their body mass index and waist-to-height ratio by 10 percent over 10 years. The later and more intense the light exposure, the worse the results.

(Interestingly, those who got the most daytime light, and the least at night, saw their weight and waist size *decrease*.)

If you can't keep electronics out of your bedroom entirely, at least shut them down an hour or so before bedtime (remember to turn off the sound on your phone or tablet) and read in soft light until you feel yourself dozing off. For those who read on a laptop or e-reading device, I recommend a free software program called f.lux (justgetflux.com). It adjusts the color of the screen to match the time of day.

No matter which you choose, closing your book or device and shutting off the light should be the last thing you remember until morning.

Wearing a sleep mask might also help if there's some light in the room (or filtering in from the outside) that you can't remove or block.

## Keep It Regular

Life doesn't always cooperate with our circadian rhythms. Some of the most sleep-deprived individuals I've met are night owls. Their bodies and minds function best at times when morning people like me are getting ready to shut it down for the night. But their jobs require them to get up early in the morning. So they lose a couple of hours of sleep every weeknight and try to make up for it by sleeping in on weekends.

Bad idea. It's possible to reset your body clock by going to bed earlier, but only if you do it consistently. A weekend is just enough time to undo whatever resetting you attempted during the week. To make it work, you need to fall asleep at the same time every night and wake up at the same time every morning.

## Create a Sleep Cave

I mentioned that your heart rate and body temperature drop in the first hour of shut-eye, when you downshift into deep sleep. A cool, quiet, clean bedroom enables the transition.

A relatively low temperature helps for the obvious reason: It's easier for you to fall into that all-important slow-wave sleep.

By "quiet," I mean devoid of erratic, unpredictable sounds, like you might get if you left the TV on. For some of us, *total* quiet actually stimulates the primitive part of the brain that learned to be very afraid when all the nocturnal creatures stop their usual nocturnal chatter. Some of us sleep better with the steady drone of a fan or the sound of rain or crickets from a bedside clock radio.

"Clean" is also relative. Dust, mold, and pet dander might not bother you when you're upright, but the minute you lay down your head, your sinuses swell up and your body struggles to get enough oxygen. And speaking of pet dander . . .

## Kick Your Pets Out of the Bedroom

Have you ever seen people try to drive with their precious Yorkie Poo or Labradoodle perched on their lap? How does the dog's presence affect their driving? If your commuting experiences are anything like mine, their speed is erratic, they struggle to stay in their lane, and they seem to have forgotten why cars have turn signals.

You can see where I'm going with this. Pets are not good bunkmates. Their sleep cycles aren't synchronized to yours. They snore. They have vivid dreams. They get up and move around. With each noise or movement, there's a non-zero chance they'll wake you up.

## Be Careful with Caffeine and Alcohol

Caffeine has a surprisingly long half-life. That cup of coffee at 3:00 p.m. may have helped you power through the final hours of work, but half of it is still in your system at 3:00 a.m. That doesn't mean you'll be awake at 3:00 a.m. If caffeine is going to interfere with your sleep, it'll do it in more subtle ways. You may not be drowsy at your normal bedtime, or you may wake up more easily, thanks to the higher level of alertness you'd expect from a stimulant.

*(continued on page 52)*

# Four Myths about Sleep

1. **Everyone needs to get 8 hours a night.** The "healthy average" is more like 7.5 hours, but even that is deceptive. Just as each of us has our own circadian rhythms, your absolute need for sleep is probably different from mine, or your spouse's, or your neighbors' or coworkers'. Whatever allows you to function at your peak—whether it's 6 hours, 9 hours, or anything in between—is what you should try to achieve.

   That said, a substantial body of research shows that sleep duration is closely linked to diabetes in a *U*-shaped pattern: The farther you get from the average of 7 to 8 hours a night, in either direction, the higher your risk for diabetes. Sleep duration by itself doesn't establish cause and effect, but if you have diabetes, your nighttime patterns can be part of the problem, and fixing them can be a big part of the solution.

2. **"My boss needs only 4 hours of sleep at night, so I shouldn't need twice that much."** Without knowing your employer, I can make a few guesses about his management style: He's a high-energy guy who can be the coolest boss ever one day and an unreasonable bastard the next. You and your coworkers are terrified of his mood swings. He gets credit for your company's successes—many of which, to be fair, result from his willingness to take risks and make out-of-the-box choices. But when one of his impulsive decisions leads to disaster, someone else gets the blame.

   So while he takes great pride in his work ethic, and boasts about how little sleep he gets as a result, your company and its employees might be better off in the hands of someone who has a more conventional schedule, makes more reasoned decisions, and manages the business less erratically. Either way, your boss's sleep patterns shouldn't interfere with yours.

3. **A nap will just keep you up at night.** This is actually true for me, but I'm a bit of an outlier. Short naps—anything from 15 to 90 minutes—have lots of

benefits. The most obvious is that a nap helps you make up for getting less sleep at night. You're more alert and better at retaining information. The naps could improve your mood, enhance your creativity, and help you avoid the late-afternoon energy crash that sends you running out for coffee and makes you crave a bag of chips. You'll be more even-tempered and less likely to blurt out something you later regret, or hit "reply all" on that e-mail with the snide comment you meant to share with just one colleague. A nap is a purge valve for the stress that builds up when you're mentally and physically fatigued.

The classic siesta takes place in the early afternoon, and that's probably the best time for it. It's the least productive part of the day for many of us, but isn't so late that it really would interfere with nighttime sleep.

4. **You shouldn't exercise too close to bedtime.** Ask me to describe the best exercise program, and I'll say it's the one you'll actually do. Ask me the best time to work out, and I'll say it's whenever you're willing to do it—within bounds of reason. A 2011 study found that young men and women got no less sleep when they did a challenging 35-minute workout 2 hours before bed, compared to a day when they didn't exercise at all. The only measurable difference was a higher heart rate during the first several hours of sleep, which would happen after a high-effort workout at any time of day. The key point is that the adrenaline generated by exercise had dissipated by bedtime.

Now, had they done the same workout at midnight, and then gone to bed immediately after, I'm sure they would've seen a different result. But that's where the "within bounds of reason" caveat comes in. Who would want to or try to fall asleep so soon after a hard run or energizing strength-training session?

As for alcohol, we think of it as a depressant, something that helps you drop off. But I've heard many stories from patients about how much better they sleep if they don't drink. My more obsessive fitness-industry friends, who sometimes track every heartbeat, marvel at how much a single drink affects their sleep quality.

I'll discuss alcohol in more detail in Chapter 7. For now, I'll just say that I enjoy an occasional drink and am not recommending abstinence. But if you think your sleep quality could be improved, you might want to stay dry for a couple of nights and see what happens.

## THINGS THAT KEEP YOU AWAKE AT NIGHT

All of us dream, and some of us dream more vividly than others. A lot of us have recurrent stress-induced dreams. About once a week I have one where I'm back in college or med school. I have a final exam, but I haven't been to class all semester, haven't cracked open the book, and sometimes can't even find the classroom. But if you're having any dreams—good or bad—consider yourself lucky, because more and more people can't fall asleep at all.

Insomnia, as a medical diagnosis, has specific criteria that can sometimes sound very much like sleep apnea: difficulty maintaining sleep, impaired performance at work or school, damaged relationships. We call it insomnia if it happens at least 3 nights a week, continues for at least 3 months, and can't be attributed to something else, like sleep-disordered breathing, a psychiatric problem such as depression, or a medical condition. Diabetes can trigger insomnia, for example, as can chronic pain or an injury that makes it uncomfortable to sleep in your normal position.

It can further be classified as transient, acute, or chronic. Transient insomnia can arise from just about any kind of illness or stress. If it continues for multiple weeks, we consider it acute, and if it lasts a month or more, it becomes chronic. At the very worst, it can trigger double vision or even hallucinations, along with the expected fatigue. That relentless exhaustion, both physical and mental, makes you more susceptible to illness and more likely to make critical or even fatal mistakes.

One easy way to tell the difference between sleep apnea and insomnia: If you struggle to fall asleep, it's probably the latter. Let's say you have money problems, or marital issues, or mounting stress at work. Or maybe you're just the type who obsesses over life's details, and right when you start to doze off, your mind replays a conversation you had with your boss. Or you realize you undertipped the waiter at Red Lobster. Or you mentally compose e-mails or texts you want to send in the morning. In an instant you go from almost asleep to fully awake, your thoughts racing and anxieties mounting. An hour later you're still awake, with something new to worry about: You're going to be a mess in the morning. It's painfully ironic when the fear of losing sleep prevents you from actually getting that sleep. (This problem is distinct from manic episodes related to bipolar disorder. In that case, you might want to work on multiple projects, with your thoughts racing both day and night, and not feel tired at all until it ends. If that happens to you, see a doctor *immediately*.)

Sleep medications like Ambien or Lunesta can be a short-term fix. But if it's a long-standing problem, you should consider cognitive behavioral therapy for insomnia (CBT-I), which is more effective for long-term relief. An experienced therapist should be able to tackle the specific problems that keep you up at night. Without therapy, and without addressing the reasons why you can't sleep, you can become dependent on the pills and suffer from rebound insomnia if you stop taking them.

# PART TWO

# EAT TO LOSE

# CHAPTER 6

# The Easiest Ways to Cut Calories

**MY CONVERSATIONS WITH PATIENTS ABOUT WEIGHT LOSS** tend to fall into three broad categories. One group, by far the smallest, includes men and women who have been trying for years to manage their weight and are often quite knowledgeable about the subject. They challenge me, in a good way, to figure out what isn't working and to come up with something that will.

A second group knows just enough about nutrition to understand that they eat way more than they should. But they're too embarrassed to admit it. The classic example is a patient with Class III obesity who tries to convince me she lives on boiled chicken breasts, undressed salads, and ice water. (When she's feeling naughty, she admits, she adds a slice of lemon.) At those moments I feel like a cop talking to a burglary suspect who denies everything, even though the stolen goods are in plain view in the backseat of his car.

But it's the third group that surprises me most, or at least used to. Unfortunately, I've worked with so many over the years that it's hard for them to say anything I haven't heard before. A typical patient in this category will describe a daily menu that includes pastries for breakfast, double and triple cheeseburgers for lunch, and pizza for dinner, washed down with 10-syllable coffee drinks, 32-ounce sodas, and a six-pack of beer.

The details change—it might be flavored teas instead of sodas, or stuffed burritos instead of burgers, or fettuccine Alfredo with bread sticks instead of pizza—but the reliance on cheap restaurant food and high-calorie beverages is consistent.

I don't know which of these patients you most resemble. My goal with this chapter is to address weight loss in a way that helps everybody. I'll start with the basics of energy balance, show some simple and (relatively) easy ways to reduce your daily calories, and then explain how to use the information to manage hunger. The next three chapters, which look at carbohydrates, protein, and fat, go into much more detail about what to eat and why. Then, in Chapters 10 and 11, I'll show how to build a sensible and sustainable diet, providing a system that you can use for as long as you want.

## WHAT IS FOOD?

Food is energy. We use it for lots of other reasons—celebration, commiseration, ritual, comfort—but to your body, it's just energy. Your body wants enough of it to get through the day without tapping into its vital reserves, which include both fat and lean tissue—muscle, bone, organs, and fluids. Both reserves increase when you eat more food than you need.

Fat is what we notice when we gain weight, but lean mass increases as well, in part to allow your body to manage the extra energy it now hordes in your fat cells. Lean tissue drives your metabolism, and your metabolism is what drives your appetite. Thus, when you get bigger, you also get hungrier, as your body wants you to eat enough to preserve your lean mass.

If you spend much time reading articles about fitness and weight loss, you probably think that muscle tissue is the most important part of your metabolism. Interestingly, it's not. Muscle uses an estimated 6 calories per pound of tissue per day, accounting for 20 to 30 percent of your resting energy expenditure, despite the fact that it makes up 40 to 50 percent of your weight. Sixty to 70 percent is burned by what researchers call high-metabolic-rate organs: the brain, heart, liver, kidneys. Your fat mass, as troublesome as it is, accounts for just 2 calories per pound per day.

Weight loss requires taking in less energy than your body needs to support its lean mass. Ideally, your body taps into your fat reserves to make up the deficit. It's like the

# METABOLISM 101

Metabolism is a series of chemical reactions that happen in every cell, all day, every day. As a technical term, it describes three things: how cells convert food into energy; how cells convert nutrients into structural tissues, like those used for muscles and bones; and how cells break down tissues to use for energy or to throw out as waste.

But when we talk about weight control, we mostly use metabolism as shorthand for *metabolic rate,* or the amount of energy we burn on an average day. It has three components.

**Resting metabolic rate (RMR):** Also called basal metabolic rate (they're not exactly the same thing, but close enough), it accounts for all the energy our bodies use just to keep us alive, which is as much as 70 percent of the calories you burn every day. RMR typically declines with age, as you lose lean mass.

**Physical activity:** Your voluntary movements—everything from walking around to fidgeting at your desk to deliberate exercise—account for about 20 percent of your daily energy use. This is the component you have the most control over.

**Thermic effect of food (TEF):** About 10 percent of your daily calories are burned digesting your meals. It's a tricky part of the equation when you're trying to lose weight, since eating less lowers your TEF. I'll address it in more detail in Chapter 8.

famous bank robber Willie Sutton allegedly said when asked why he robs banks: "Because that's where the money is." Fat is your body's energy vault, providing 3,500 calories per pound, enough to get most of us through an entire day. Muscle tissue, on the other hand, offers very little energy. A pound of muscle has 454 grams of protein, about 1,800 calories' worth, which your body must first convert to glucose.

But losing a lot of weight inevitably means losing some lean tissue along with the fat. Some of the loss will come from muscle, partly because your body will use it for energy, and partly because you simply don't need as much muscle when there's so much less weight to haul around. You'll even lose a tiny amount from those high-metabolic-rate organs, which are now part of a smaller organism. The loss of lean tissue will slow your metabolism, as will the fact that you're eating less food.

I'll address some of these issues in the diet and workout chapters. For now, if you're at the beginning of a weight-loss program, your goal is to make the simplest, easiest adjustments, most of which shouldn't affect your metabolism in any major way.

## THE FIRST (AND MOST IMPORTANT) STEPS

When you eat something typically described with a modifier like "fast," "packaged," or "convenience," you're getting food that's been deliberately manipulated with sugar, fat, and salt to make it more appetizing. If it tastes better, you'll eat more of it. You'll eat when you aren't hungry, and continue eating long after you should've stopped. As I mentioned in Chapter 3, your body's defenses against overeating don't stand a chance against food engineered to bypass them.

So your first step, logically, is to avoid that kind of food whenever you can. Specifically:

- Prepare as many meals as possible at home.

- When you prepare those meals, try to build them around fresh plant and animal foods.

- When you use packaged ingredients, look at the labels and try to avoid the ones with the most added sugar, fat, and salt.

- Avoid anything deep-fried: french fries, onion rings, chicken nuggets, mozzarella sticks, chips, breaded fish or meat, calamari, egg rolls, dumplings . . .

- Wherever you eat—home, work, restaurants, or in transit from one to another—avoid liquid calories from soda, juice, or flavored tea. Diet versions of those drinks are acceptable.

- Coffee is great, except when it turns into coffee-flavored dessert. If you need to add flavor, choose artificial sweeteners and low-calorie creamers.

- Avoid distracted eating. Try not to eat at your desk or in front of the TV, both of which are linked to eating more.

- Drink a glass of water before each meal. Your stomach has only so much room. Filling part of it with water leaves less room for food, and you'll feel full faster.

And here's one more tip that works for every patient of mine who tries it: *Take a walk after dinner.* Or after lunch. Or after any meal, really. On top of the handful of calories it burns, research shows that it helps lower blood sugar levels in people with type 2 diabetes. It's also one of the most *social* weight-loss methods you'll find. You can disconnect from electronic entertainment and reconnect with your spouse and/or kids. Stop and chat with neighbors. Give the dog a chance to sniff something interesting.

Don't worry about how far you go or how fast you get there. Fifteen to 20 minutes on your feet—and away from the temptation to eat more—are all it takes.

## FIX YOUR ENVIRONMENT FOR LONG-LASTING EFFECTS

The tips in the previous section all help, but they work only when you use them. A few simple changes to your kitchen and dining areas help you use them more often. Many of these tips come from *Mindless Eating* and *Slim by Design,* both by Brian

Wansink, PhD, a behavioral scientist and founder of the Cornell University Food and Brand Lab.

## Manage Your Line of Sight

Temptation begins with the eyes, and what you see is what you'll eat, sooner or later. Dr. Wansink's research shows that if you hide packaged foods (like breakfast cereal) behind cabinet doors, instead of leaving them out on countertops, you won't be tempted to eat them for a snack. The same advice holds for your office: Keep food hidden in drawers, cabinets, or a refrigerator.

Another simple but crucial change: When you're eating a family dinner, put salads on the table, but leave the main course back in the kitchen, or at least off the table and out of reach. You're much less likely to have a second helping when you have to get up from the table to get it.

On the flip side, you want healthy foods in plain view. If you have a candy dish, replace it with a bowl of fruit. You'll eat more fruit and fewer sweets—a double win.

## Think Small

If you could transport yourself back 50 years to a holiday dinner at a grandparent's house, one of the first things you'd notice is how much smaller the plates, glasses, and silverware were. The plates your parents' parents used for dinner were about the size of today's salad plates. Same with cutlery: A dinner fork back then might be smaller than a salad fork in a restaurant today, and I think many of us would struggle to finish a bowl of chowder using one of Grandma's soup spoons. Ours are like garden tools by comparison. But perhaps the biggest upward growth is with our glassware. If your grandparents saw a wine glass in one of today's more elegant restaurants, they might think it was a long-stemmed fishbowl. Their glasses were designed to hold 4 to 5 ounces. Even half-filled, ours hold twice that much.

You probably think that smaller plates just make you hungry for seconds, but it doesn't actually work that way. When Dr. Wansink's test subjects downsized from 12- to 10-inch dinner plates, they ate proportionally less food. Another experiment showed that bartenders serve more when they use shorter, wider glasses, instead of taller, narrower ones.

Size also matters when you're buying food in bulk. The more you buy, the more you'll eat. That applies not only to Sam's Club and Costco, but also to restaurants and movie theaters. If you buy anything billed as "bottomless" or promising free refills, chances are pretty good you'll take them up on that offer, and put away hundreds of calories you didn't expect or even want.

But wait a second: If you weren't hungry, why did you eat it? That's a question worth exploring.

## THE HUNGER GAME

If your body could be perfectly calibrated, any hunger you felt would drive you to eat just enough food to match your physiological needs. So if you exercised a little more one day, you'd be a little hungrier, and eat a little more. If you got a *lot* more activity, you would be a *lot* hungrier, and eat a *lot* more. And if you spent the weekend in bed binge-watching all seven seasons of *Mad Men,* your appetite would drop accordingly (give or take a martini or two).

It's a beautiful idea, but real life is too complicated for that. Your energy intake has never been, and will never be, 100 percent correlated to your energy expenditure. So in the absence of perfection, your body improvises. Most people eat a little less on workdays, somewhat more on weekends, and quite a bit more on holidays. After a couple days of eating less than usual, or moving more than usual, your appetite should pick up to close the deficit. The same thing should happen in reverse when you overdo it for a couple of days: You should be less hungry for a day or two while your body deals with the excess.

Obesity and diabetes disrupt this bias toward equilibrium. Fat, as I've explained, develops a mind of its own, and your body builds resistance to key hormones that regulate appetite. Regaining control over your hunger is a meal-by-meal struggle that hinges on two processes with similar names but different meanings.

*Satiation* is the feeling that you are full and don't need to eat any more at that particular meal. It's partly based on volume: In between meals, your stomach may hold about 2 fluid ounces. It rapidly expands when you eat and drink, holding a maximum of 2 to 4 liters (68 to 135 ounces), although you should feel full long before then. Stomach expansion sends signals to your brain to stop eating. And it's partly based on time, which is why eating slower usually means eating less. The more time you give your body to take inventory of what you've eaten, and how much, the less total food you'll need in that meal.

*Satiety* determines how much time elapses between meals before you start getting hungry again. It's influenced partly by the number of calories in the most recent meal and partly by the composition of the meal. Fiber and protein generally lead to more satiety. Highly processed foods—white bread, pastries, sweets—provide the least. Soda offers virtually none at all.

Both processes are flavor-specific. The more choices you have, the more you'll eat. Imagine a steak dinner. You might eat 6 to 8 ounces and feel happy and full. But then someone offers ice cream or cheesecake, and all of a sudden you're hungry again.

Hunger control is the key to weight control. And the key to hunger control is situational management. You know that fast food is engineered to make it as easy as possible to eat as much as possible, so you avoid fast food. You know that snack foods are processed with sugar, fat, and salt with the goal of making you hungrier for snack foods, so you don't bring them into your home or office. You know that variety expands your appetite for different flavors, so you limit the number of choices you have available to you.

So what should those choices be, and how should you make them? That's what we'll cover in the next four chapters.

## CHAPTER 7

# Straight Talk about Carbohydrates

**WHEN I STARTED PRACTICING MEDICINE,** I was completely sold on low-carb diets. They worked for me, and when I treated patients with diabetes, my gut told me that the fewer carbs they ate, the faster they would reverse the disease. Logically, a low-carb diet should connect all the dots.

- Diabetes begins with insulin resistance. The normal amount of insulin no longer gets food out of your bloodstream and into your cells.

- Insulin resistance causes high blood sugar—essentially, a backlog of glucose waiting to get into cells. Your pancreas responds by cranking out more insulin.

- The sugar in your blood comes primarily from carbohydrates in your meals. The more carbs you eat, the higher your blood sugar goes, and the more insulin you produce to get rid of it.

- If you eat fewer carbs, you'll have less blood sugar.

- If you have less blood sugar, your body doesn't need to produce as much insulin.

- Eventually, as your insulin and glucose levels decline, your sensitivity to insulin should return to normal.

Does it work that well in practice? Among my patients, yes, but only if they can stick with it. If more of them could, I'd try to get all of them on low-carb diets. Adherence is almost always the biggest challenge for my patients. It's a problem that shows up pretty consistently in research as well. Researchers have compared a long list of diets, from super-low-carb to super-low-fat, and lots in between, and found little compelling evidence that any one diet is superior to the others for improving the symptoms of diabetes. (For patients whose diabetes is more advanced, it's a different story. I encourage *much* lower carbs, as I explain in Chapter 10.)

But as my friends who publish studies like to say, absence of evidence isn't evidence of absence. (They also like to say, "The plural of 'anecdote' isn't 'data.'" And yet, against all odds, they're fun to hang out with.) Diabetes is a really difficult disease to study because it has so many moving parts. If a diet is shown to help lower blood sugar, but it also helps volunteers lose weight, how do you know what was cause and what was effect? Did blood sugar go down because of the diet, or because of the weight loss? And if it's because of the weight loss—because the subjects ate less food, in other words—how do we know this is the *best* diet for that goal? Medications are also wild cards. If someone's blood sugar didn't change, but she was able to use lower doses, does that mean the diet was successful?

Another problem is adherence. If you sign up for a study, you don't get to pick your own diet. Through a process called randomization, the researchers choose one for you. Imagine that you're a lifelong meat eater, and you get randomized to a low-fat vegan diet. Or you're someone who loves your cereal in the morning and a sandwich for lunch, but you get assigned to a low-carb diet that eliminates most of your favorite foods. How would you react? You might give it an honest try for a month or two, but eventually you'd wander back to the way you prefer to eat. That's a huge problem in many diet studies; the researchers have to trust that their volunteers will eat the way they're told.

So it's entirely possible that if most of the subjects were able to stick to their assigned diets, they'd show clear differences. That is, some would be demonstrably superior.

But on the third hand, would it really matter? If the diets are so unpalatable that very few people are able to stick to them, is there any benefit in knowing that one might be better than the others?

I know this is a long intro, but these are important questions about a controversial topic. My patients who've done their homework have more questions about carbohydrates than anything else related to nutrition. The ones trying to lose weight have gotten more conflicting advice. Even doctors can't agree. The debates might be more polite in medical journals than they are online, but if you know how to read between the lines, you see they're just as passionate. So I wanted to start this chapter by making it clear that I'm not taking a militant stance on either side of the argument, and I'm especially not recommending an extreme diet.

With that out of the way, let's start with a fundamental question that a surprising number of my patients are confused about.

## WHAT IS A CARBOHYDRATE?

A carbohydrate is one of the three macronutrients, or energy nutrients. The other two, of course, are fat and protein. (Alcohol earns a separate designation, as you'll see in "What about Booze?" on page 74.) In a typical American diet, carbs provide as many calories as the other two combined. They come almost exclusively from plant foods, with the exception of milk and dairy products. You can divide them into two categories: sugars and starches. (Fibers are technically a third category, which I'll get to later in this chapter.)

### Sugars

Sugars are often described as "simple" carbs, which is accurate enough if you're just looking at the chemistry. But when a dietitian gets on the radio and tells everyone to avoid all simple carbs, the term becomes misleading at best. The category includes everything from table sugar to fruit, vegetables, and milk.

There's little reason to fear the ones that occur in nature, unless you're intolerant to lactose, the sugar found in dairy. Fruits are loaded with sugars, as are corn, bell peppers, and root vegetables like beets, carrots, and onions. Then there's honey, which is pure sugar (and the only natural carbohydrate I tell my patients to avoid entirely). Proponents of "ancestral" diets often claim that pre-agricultural humans ate a low-carb diet, and certainly some of them did, but not by choice. Anthropologists who study the few remaining hunter-gatherer tribes note that they gladly consume honey whenever and wherever they find it. Same with super-sweet fruits like berries.

The foods I mentioned contain various amounts of three sugars: glucose, fructose, and sucrose, which is a combination of the first two. Table sugar is pure sucrose. What we call high-fructose corn syrup is just sucrose with a slightly higher percentage of fructose. There's not much functional difference among these sugars. They're all easy to overeat, and their calories add up quickly.

## By Any Other Name...

The following is a partial list of the many names for sugar that's added to food. (I've left out the obvious ones, like cane sugar, that don't make you guess what they are.)

- Agave nectar
- Barley malt syrup
- Caramel
- Corn syrup
- Dextrose
- Fructose
- Galactose
- Glucose
- High-fructose corn syrup
- Honey
- Lactose
- Maltose
- Maple syrup
- Molasses
- Sucrose

## Starches

Starches are alternately praised (because they're "complex" carbohydrates) and demonized (because they're carbs). But in truth it's too broad a category for black-and-white judgments. Major sources of starch include:

- Grains (wheat, corn, rice, oats, barley)

- Tubers (potatoes, yams, sweet potatoes)

- Legumes (peas, lentils, beans, peanuts, soybeans)

- Starchy vegetables (pumpkin, squash)

As a housekeeping note, the category of "starchy vegetables" is often expanded by dietitians to include legumes, tubers, and even corn (which, as I noted, is a grain). I like to keep them separate to emphasize the differences in fiber and protein. Almost all starches are broken down into glucose and sent into your bloodstream, but those with the least fiber and protein get there fastest and create the biggest spike in post-meal blood sugar. That's the subject of our next section.

## GLYCEMIC INDEX VERSUS GLYCEMIC LOAD

On the day you were diagnosed with diabetes, or with prediabetes, or simply told that you have high blood sugar, you were probably given a handout describing the glycemic index (GI). So most of you already know that it's a measure of how fast different foods are digested and sent into your bloodstream.

At the high end of the scale, with a GI of 100, is 50 grams of pure glucose. At the opposite end are foods like beef, walnuts, avocado, and celery, which have virtually no carbohydrates and therefore a GI of zero. A GI of 70 or above is considered high; low is 55 or below. Here are a few examples.

# GLYCEMIC INDEX

| FOOD | GI |
|------|-----|
| Baked potato | 85 |
| Popcorn | 72 |
| Watermelon | 72 |
| White bread | 70 |
| Table sugar (sucrose) | 68 |
| Mac 'n' cheese | 64 |
| White rice | 64 |
| Ice cream | 61 |
| Oatmeal | 58 |
| Brown rice | 55 |
| Snickers bar | 55 |
| Banana | 52 |
| Carrots | 47 |
| Apple | 38 |
| Pizza | 30 |
| Peanuts | 14 |

If you went by the GI, and nothing else, you might conclude that potatoes are more dangerous than table sugar, a Snickers bar is better than oatmeal, and pizza looks healthier than carrots. That's one big problem with GI: It's based on a uniform serving size equal to 50 grams of carbohydrates. Fifty grams of carrots is 4½ cups. Even for Bugs Bunny that's a bit excessive.

But it's not the only problem. GI can vary by up to 50 percent from one person to the next. Even for the same person, it might vary at different times and in different circumstances. For example, if you complete an exhausting workout, or a long hike, your muscles will be drained of glycogen. Higher-carb foods will have a lower GI because your muscles are so receptive to the glucose they put into your bloodstream.

The serving size issue led researchers to create another scale: glycemic load (GL). This one estimates the amount of glucose that would reach your bloodstream based on a typical serving size. To calculate GL, you divide GI by 100, and then multiply by "net carbohydrates"—grams of carbs minus grams of fiber, since humans can't turn dietary fiber into energy.

Unfortunately, that leaves us with two completely different scales. A high GL is 20 or above; low is 10 or below. Here's what they look like side by side.

## GLYCEMIC INDEX VERSUS GLYCEMIC LOAD

| FOOD | GI | GL (SERVING SIZE) |
|---|---|---|
| Baked potato | 85 | 28 (1 medium) |
| Popcorn | 72 | 7 (2 cups) |
| Watermelon | 72 | 8 (1 cup) |
| White bread | 70 | 10 (1 slice) |
| Table sugar (sucrose) | 68 | 8 (1 tablespoon) |
| Mac 'n' cheese | 64 | 30 (1 serving) |
| White rice | 64 | 33 (1 cup) |
| Ice cream | 61 | 10 (1 cup) |
| Oatmeal | 58 | 12 (1 cup) |
| Brown rice | 55 | 23 (1 cup) |
| Snickers bar | 55 | 35 (4-oz King Size bar) |
| Banana | 52 | 14 (1 large) |
| Carrots | 47 | 2 (1 large) |
| Apple | 38 | 6 (1 medium) |
| Pizza | 30 | 13 (2 slices) |
| Peanuts | 14 | <1 (¼ cup) |

You can quibble over whether those are typical serving sizes. Some might be a lot less than you'd actually consume, and that's really important. Take white bread, for example. Since you need two slices to make a sandwich, the GL doubles from 10 to 20.

The big point about glycemic load is this: For someone with diabetes, a lower GL is better. But how are you supposed to know the exact GL of any given meal? Do you carry a guidebook everywhere you go? Or boot up a smartphone app for every meal?

Both can work, if you have that kind of discipline. If you don't, here's a good rule of thumb.

*Limit yourself to 40 grams of net carbs per meal, and 20 per snack.*

Now you've made it simple. A nutrition label will tell you how many grams of carbs there are per serving, and how much fiber. Subtract the fiber from the carbs to get net carbs per serving. And then multiply by however many servings you expect to eat.

But what if there isn't a label to consult? These tips should help you avoid a large GL.

- Avoid sugar-rich beverages—soda, specialty coffees and teas, and juices. (I'm surprised at how few of my patients realize that fruit juice is 100 percent sugar.) The same goes for alcoholic drinks that arrive in punch bowls, like a mai tai.

- Avoid meals that are all or mostly carbs, like sandwiches on kaiser rolls or platters of pasta. Especially avoid carbs on top of carbs by having bread with your pasta.

- With any carb-based entrée, like a sandwich or pizza, go for the thinnest bread slices or crust. Whole wheat is probably better than white, although I often suspect it's the same thing, only with caramel coloring.

- If you make pasta at home, have it al dente, or slightly undercooked. That leaves some of the starch indigestible, which means it won't contribute to the GL.

- Include some protein in every meal. I'll go into all of this in great detail in Chapter 8, but for now just keep in mind that protein doesn't have any glycemic index or load.

- The same goes for fat—no GI or GL. I'll explain in Chapter 9 which fats are best for you.

That brings us to the final tip, and perhaps the most important point I'll make about carbohydrates: The best carbs are the ones with lots of fiber.

# FIBER IS YOUR FRIEND

Any good diet should do four essential things.

1. Give you a structured way to eat less

2. Reduce the amount of prepared food you eat, and increase the number of meals you cook or put together at home

3. Emphasize whole foods over those that are processed and packaged

4. Increase fiber

Of those, the first is the most important, since it allows you to lose weight—usually the key selling point to any popular diet. The next two are what make it possible. And fiber, to quote The Dude from *The Big Lebowski,* is what ties the whole room together. It's the common link between low-carb paleo and low-fat vegan: Both emphasize plant foods (to the exclusion of animal foods, in the vegan diet), and both provide a *lot* more fiber than the average person gets in a day.

In experimental studies with volunteers who have diabetes, those who got more fiber usually decreased both fasting blood sugar and hemoglobin A1C. In large epidemiological studies—those that compile data on what people do, or at least recall doing, and correlate behaviors with outcomes—the ones who habitually consume the most fiber have dramatically lower rates of heart disease. We also know that higher fiber consumption is linked to a lower risk of having diabetes in the first place.

There's a lot of upside to increasing dietary fiber, and virtually no downside, unless you have digestive issues. Foods that are relatively high in fiber—whole grains, fruits, vegetables, legumes—are associated with a lower risk of just about every major disease. It's impossible to say if that's because of fiber alone, or because of some combination of vitamins, minerals, and fiber that occurs naturally in plants, but not in highly processed versions of those foods. When in doubt, always choose whole grains over refined, and whole fruits and vegetables over juices.

So let's talk numbers.

*(continued on page 76)*

# WHAT ABOUT BOOZE?

Alcohol has a prominent role in medical and political history, not to mention the annals of crime and punishment. As Homer Simpson once said, when proposing a toast, "To alcohol! The cause of, and solution to, all of life's problems!" Our genes for metabolizing alcohol go back millions of years, to a time when extremely ancient hominids discovered they could get a buzz from eating rotten fruit that had fermented in the warm, humid forest. (Its potency is equivalent to an average beer.) So ingrained is alcohol in human history, in fact, that we've been making it as long as we've been growing crops that we could make it from.

You've probably heard that moderate alcohol consumption—an average of two drinks a day for men, one a day for women—offers health benefits, which is true. Studies have shown that it lowers the risk of developing type 2 diabetes by 20 percent in men and a whopping 43 percent in women. The effect is strongest in those 60 and older, and in those with a family history of the disease when compared to those without.

We also know that moderate drinking is associated with lower cardiovascular disease rates and overall mortality risk. This applies to those with diabetes as well as those without.

Doctors like me have traditionally told patients that a little alcohol is okay if it's something you do anyway, but if you don't drink, there's no reason to start. We now know that last part may not be true. A recent study in *Annals of Internal Medicine* had non-drinking volunteers take up the habit with 5 ounces a night of either red or white wine. Red wine increased HDL cholesterol and reduced the risk of metabolic syndrome. White wine reduced fasting blood glucose.

So I'm all about the alcohol now, right?

No.

First off, I've had lots of patients who tell me they drink an entire bottle of wine or case of beer a night. That's full-on alcoholism, and the risk of that overshadows the potential benefits of moderate drinking. But my biggest concern for both moderate and heavy drinkers is the effect on your weight.

Alcohol has 7 calories per gram, which puts it somewhere between protein and carbs (4 calories) and fat (9 calories). But your body doesn't like having alcohol in your system. It's not an essential nutrient, and it can't be stored. So you metabolize alcohol immediately and preferentially, which means anything you eat goes to the back of the line while your body gets rid of the booze.

Here's why that's a problem.

The term "beer goggles" applies to more than your mating decisions at closing time. Alcohol has a profound effect on your food choices. Your inhibition drops and your intake increases. Where do those calories go? They're *much* more likely to be stored as fat.

I don't mean to come off as a scold. I enjoy an occasional drink, as do most of my friends. Research shows genuine health benefits within specific parameters. If you enjoy a glass of wine with your dinner or like to unwind with a beer after work, and can stay within those limits, there's good reason to believe you'll live a longer life, with less risk of heart disease. But if you're consistently drinking three or four times that much, it would probably be a good idea to cut back.

The average American adult gets about 15 grams of fiber a day, or 7 grams for every 1,000 calories. Most health organizations recommend at least 14 grams per 1,000 calories, or 25 grams a day for women and 38 for men. Those aren't magic numbers, but when it comes to nutrition, nothing is. All I can say for certain is that almost everyone I see in my practice undershoots those targets. The ones who increase their fiber consumption lose weight and see their health improve in multiple ways.

## FIBER-RICH FOODS

| FOOD | SERVING | FIBER (GRAMS) |
|---|---|---|
| Legumes | | |
| Navy beans, cooked from dried | ½ cup | 9.6 |
| Split peas, cooked from dried | ½ cup | 8.1 |
| Lentils, cooked from dried | ½ cup | 7.8 |
| Black beans, canned | ½ cup | 7.5 |
| Kidney beans, canned | ½ cup | 6.8 |
| Cereals and Grains | | |
| Kashi GoLean cereal | 1¼ cups | 13 |
| Kellogg's All-Bran cereal | ½ cup | 10 |
| Quinoa, cooked | 1 cup | 5.2 |
| Oatmeal, cooked | 1 cup | 4.0 |
| Brown rice, medium grain, cooked | 1 cup | 3.5 |
| Corn on the cob | 1 medium | 2.9 |
| Whole wheat bread | 1 slice | 1.9 |
| Vegetables | | |
| Artichoke hearts, cooked | ½ cup | 7.2 |
| Broccoli, cooked | 1 medium stalk | 5.9 |
| Spinach, frozen, cooked | ½ cup | 3.5 |
| Green beans | 1 cup | 3.4 |
| Brussels sprouts, frozen, cooked | ½ cup | 3.2 |

| | | |
|---|---|---|
| Winter squash, cooked | 1 cup | 2.9 |
| Cauliflower, cooked | 1 cup | 2.8 |
| Mushrooms, white, cooked from fresh | 1 cup | 1.7 |
| Fruits | | |
| Prunes, uncooked | ½ cup, pitted | 6.2 |
| Pear | 1 medium | 5.5 |
| Guava, fresh | ½ cup | 4.5 |
| Apple | 1 medium | 4.4 |
| Orange | 1 large | 4.4 |
| Raspberries, fresh | ½ cup | 4.0 |
| Blackberries, fresh | ½ cup | 3.8 |
| Banana | 1 medium | 3.1 |
| Nuts and Seeds | | |
| Almonds | 1 ounce (23 nuts) | 3.5 |
| Pistachio nuts | 1 ounce (49 nuts) | 2.9 |
| Pecans | 1 ounce (19 halves) | 2.7 |
| Peanuts | 1 ounce (about ¼ cup) | 2.4 |

Adapted from *The Lean Muscle Diet* (Rodale, 2014) by Lou Schuler and Alan Aragon

# FINAL THOUGHTS ABOUT CARBS

I started this chapter by saying I used to be a huge advocate of low-carb diets, and I mean that literally: I weighed 265 pounds in my final season as a college wrestler. My low-carb diet helped me drop 30 pounds. But when I decided to compete again—first in bodybuilding, then in triathlon—I switched over to a higher-carb, lower-fat diet, keeping protein the same. I was surprised by how much better I felt, and how much more energy I had for my workouts. This doesn't mean much for my patients, or for you, except that it reinforced an important truth about nutrition: There are lots of ways to achieve the same goals—to lose weight, to lower your blood sugar, and to improve your odds for a longer, healthier life.

You can accomplish all that with a low-carb diet that includes a lot of meat, a low-fat vegetarian or vegan diet, or the modified Mediterranean diet that I describe in Chapter 10. As long as it allows you to eat less food and still exercise as much and as energetically as you want, just about any diet will get you to the same place.

When it comes to carbs specifically, I think there are really just four rules for those who have diabetes or know they're at risk of developing it. The first is the one I mentioned earlier.

1. *Limit yourself to 40 net grams of carbs per meal, and 20 per snack.* Remember: "Net carbs" are total grams of carbs minus grams of fiber. The next three rules come into play when you can't tally up net carbs easily or accurately.

2. *Avoid the most highly processed grain-based foods,* especially those you'll typically eat way too much of, like pancakes and waffles, pastries, pizza, pasta, and sandwiches that test the range of motion of your jaws.

3. *Avoid high-sugar beverages entirely.* There's absolutely no benefit to drinking sodas, flavored coffees and teas, juices, and alcoholic drinks made with any of those things.

4. *Remember that fiber-rich carbs have amazing benefits.* Any time you can replace processed or prepared foods with whole foods high in fiber, you're doing something positive for your health.

If you're wondering how you're going to get along without some of your favorite foods, there's a simple answer: Eat more protein, the subject of the next chapter.

## CHAPTER 8

# The Power of Protein

**ADDING MORE PROTEIN TO YOUR DIET** is possibly the most effective change you can make for both weight loss and diabetes management. It offers three huge benefits.

- Protein increases both satiation (you feel full sooner while eating) and satiety (you're full longer between meals).

- Protein has a higher thermic effect. About 25 percent of its energy is burned off during digestion, compared to about 6 to 8 percent for carbs and 2 to 3 percent for fat.

- Protein helps preserve lean mass when you're trying to lose weight, and it helps you build muscle in the context of a workout program.

Put them all together, and here's what you get by eating more protein.

- Because it fills you up faster, and makes you feel full longer, you eat less overall food.

- Because of the high thermic effect, less of the food you eat will be available as energy.

- Eating more protein generally means eating less of everything else at any given meal, which leaves you with less sugar and fat in your bloodstream, and thus better glycemic control.

- The combination of these benefits leads to weight loss, with more of that weight from fat.

- If you're training for strength, you'll build some new muscle, or at minimum improve your muscle quality while losing fat and preserving lean tissue.

But perhaps the best and most underrated benefit of eating more protein is that it's nearly impossible for your body to turn it into fat. To understand why, we have to start with the most basic question.

## WHAT IS PROTEIN?

Along with carbohydrate and fat, protein is a macronutrient. But it's the one your body is least likely to use for energy. Even during a really long exercise bout—a day-long hike, say, or a 100-mile bike ride—your body might get 10 percent of its energy from protein. The rest will come preferentially from carbs while they're plentiful, and then from fat.

So what happens to the protein in your diet? Your body has lots of ways to use it. About 20 percent of your body is made of protein, which doesn't sound like much until you consider that 60 to 65 percent is water. So in a lean individual 20 percent represents the majority of his body's dry mass. Even in someone with obesity, muscle might be equal to fat as a percentage of non-water weight, or nearly so. Forty percent of your body's protein is stored in your muscles, 25 percent in your organs, and the rest primarily in your skin, hair, and blood. Structural proteins hold your body together, while unbound proteins—including hormones, enzymes, and anti-bodies—send signals that tell every part of your body what to do, and how to do it.

The protein you can't store is converted to glucose and used for energy. In theory, *some* of it could be converted to fat, but I can't imagine a circumstance in which this would occur. You'd have to eat thousands of calories' worth of protein, which would be absurdly difficult given the appetite-blunting effects of normal amounts. Then you have the thermic effect, with a quarter of the calories burning off in digestion.

Here's why that's important.

We all overeat sometimes—weekends, holidays, parties. When it happens, your body has a few different ways of dealing with the excess energy. It burns some off during digestion. You may also engage in more spontaneous physical activity. That is, you move around more without planning to, or even noticing. You feel more energetic because you literally have more energy to burn.

What you don't burn off in digestion or by fidgeting or puttering around, you'll store. Now, if those excess calories are from fat, you can store it pretty easily in your fat cells, where there's plenty of room. The process is more complicated for carbohydrate—your body prefers to use it for energy—but because there are so few places to store it, and because those places have such limited capacity, your body converts the carbs to triglycerides and tucks them away in your fat cells.

Protein is different.

You can see why protein is so valuable when you're trying to lose weight and reduce blood sugar. But for long-term health, its effect on your muscle tissue may be even more valuable.

## IF YOU BUILD IT . . .

Muscle cells add and subtract protein throughout the day. The build-up process—*anabolism*—accelerates at two times: right after you eat, and after a challenging workout. Protein breakdown—*catabolism*—sounds like something you want to avoid. But in truth it's crucial for your health because it gets rid of older, malformed, and dysfunctional cells so they can be replaced by new ones. When you're young and growing, the net effect is that you end up with more protein in your muscles. Through early adulthood you probably break even. And then, starting in middle age, the overall balance is negative. You lose some muscle each year, and the more you lose, the easier it is to store fat. Over time, the combined effects of age, inactivity, and lower muscle quality leave you in a state of *anabolic resistance,* with your muscles storing less of the protein from your meals.

Let's go back to the idea of your body as a factory. But instead of focusing on the loading docks, as we did in Chapter 2, we'll go deeper inside, to the machines that keep everything up and running. These machines require a lot of maintenance, including a fresh supply of spare parts every few hours or so. Which, yes, would be a very odd business model for a factory, but it doesn't matter because we're just pretending. As the machines get older, they require more spare parts to do the same job. Unless you increase the volume of parts coming into your factory, you'll lose more machines as they go offline. The longer a machine sits dormant, the harder it is to get it working again.

That's the effect of anabolic resistance. The solution is straightforward enough: more protein in your meals. Research leads us to a precise number: 30 grams per meal. That amount works better for both satiety and anabolism, when compared against smaller amounts.

But there are two pretty important conditions.

1. It has to be high-quality protein.

2. It has to be eaten in at least three meals a day.

## QUALITY

Nature makes protein molecules by mixing and matching 20 different amino acids, some of which are far more potent for building muscle. Animal foods—meat, fish, poultry, eggs, dairy—are considered the highest-quality protein sources because they offer the most concentrated volumes of those potent amino acids. Legumes like soybeans, lentils, and black beans are also good sources. But because the protein is less concentrated in most of them (soybeans are an exception), you need to eat more of those foods to reach 30 grams. Grains have even less.

This chart shows how to get to that 30-gram threshold from a variety of sources. The examples are pretty absurd when you get to the bottom of the list (like a half-cup of peanut butter, or 12 slices of bread), and I'm definitely not recommending them. I just want to show how some foods can help you reach the threshold all by themselves, while others contribute relatively little protein to a meal.

| FOOD | SERVING SIZE* | PROTEIN (GRAMS) | 30 GRAMS† |
|---|---|---|---|
| Chicken breast | ½ breast | 30 | ½ breast |
| Soybeans | 1 cup | 29 | 1 cup |
| Cottage cheese | 1 cup | 28 | 1 cup |
| Salmon | 4 ounces | 23 | 5 ounces |
| Beef (sirloin) | 4 ounces | 21 | 6 ounces |
| Greek yogurt | 1 cup | 20 | 1½ cups |
| Shrimp | 3 ounces | 17 | 5 ounces |
| Chicken thigh | 1 thigh | 16 | 2 thighs |
| Lentils | 1 cup | 16 | 2 cups |
| Brown rice | 1 cup | 15 | 2 cups |
| Black beans | 1 cup | 15 | 2 cups |
| Wild rice | ½ cup | 13 | 1 cup+ |
| Eggs | 2 eggs | 12 | 5 eggs |
| Milk (2%) | 1 cup | 8 | 4 cups |
| Peanut butter | 2 tablespoons | 8 | ½ cup |
| Mozzarella cheese (part skim) | 1 ounce | 7 | 4 ounces |
| Cashews | ¼ cup | 5 | 1½ cups |
| Whole wheat bread | 2 slices | 5 | 12 slices |

*This is a typical serving size, which may be more or less than you would actually eat.

†This is the volume of food needed to get close to 30 grams. To keep the math simple, it may end up a couple of grams over or under.

# Meals

In a typical eating pattern, you get as much as two-thirds of your daily protein with dinner. You probably have very little protein at breakfast, if you eat breakfast at all. Lots of people simply aren't hungry in the morning, including some whose stomachs would take sadistic turns if they tried to force anything down. For others, breakfast is just one more thing to do, and on most days they choose not to do it. Then there are those—including some of my patients—who skip it with the goal of losing weight.

I could pull out data showing that people who eat breakfast are leaner, lighter, live longer, and have better-behaved children, compared to those who skip it. But I don't, in part because I just made up the thing about kids. Mainly, though, I don't push breakfast on non-breakfast eaters for the same reason I don't pressure patients to go on extreme diets or eat foods they find unappealing. I've rarely seen that kind of program work. But I've seen plenty of patients lose weight and improve their health—sometimes in dramatic ways—with diets built around foods they like and eating patterns they can live with. If that includes breakfast, great. If not, just substitute the phrase "my first meal of the day" whenever I mention breakfast. Time is just a number, right? (Okay, not when your boss expects you in the office at 9:00 a.m., but you know what I mean.)

Whatever you call it, *any* meal in the morning leaves you feeling fuller throughout the day, with fewer food cravings. A higher-protein breakfast increases those benefits, to the point that volunteers in studies snacked less in the evening, compared to those who'd started their day with a lower-protein meal. You don't seem to get any of those benefits from the same amount of protein at lunch or dinner.

Of course it's easy to get 30 grams of protein at lunch or dinner—you can pick anything from the top half of the chart I just showed you, or mix and match a few of the items from the middle of the list. A cup of lentils and a cup of brown rice, combined in an appetizing way, get you there pretty easily. But how do you get 30 grams of protein from your first meal of the day?

The chart opposite gives you some cornerstones of a traditional breakfast (eggs, cereal, cottage cheese) and a few suggestions for foods that might go well with them. Some of them have protein (milk, cheese, nuts), some don't (fruits and vegetables). Disregard my suggestions if you see more appetizing ways to reach the right amount.

| START WITH . . . | PROTEIN (GRAMS) | COMBINE WITH (PROTEIN GRAMS) . . . |
|---|---|---|
| 3 eggs (omelet or scrambled) | 18 | · 2 ounces ham (10)<br>· 2 slices whole wheat toast (5)<br>· 1 ounce mozzarella cheese (7)<br>· Fresh vegetables (n/a) |
| 1½ scoops whey protein | 30* | · Fresh fruit in a smoothie (n/a) |
| 1 cup cottage cheese | 28 | · ¼ cup chopped walnuts (4)<br>· Fresh fruit (n/a) |
| 1 cup Greek yogurt | 20 | · ¼ cup sliced almonds (7)<br>· Fresh fruit (n/a) |
| 1¼ cups Kashi GoLean cereal | 12 | · 1 cup 2% milk (8)<br>· 1 hard-cooked egg (8) |
| 1 cup oatmeal | 6 | · 1 scoop vanilla protein powder (20*)<br>· 1 tablespoon chia seeds (2)<br>· Fresh fruit (n/a) |
| 3 ounces smoked salmon | 15 | · ½ cup Greek yogurt (10)<br>· 2 slices whole wheat toast (5) |

*Different brands use different quantities per scoop. Choose whatever gets you to 30 grams for the meal.*

## WARNINGS, REAL VERSUS UNWARRANTED

I can't talk about protein without a few words about safety. It's an article of faith among many of my colleagues that protein is dangerous, with the potential to damage kidneys and weaken bones. Sometimes they pass these warnings along to patients, teaching them to be afraid of a nutrient that can help them in all the ways I just described.

To be fair, there is a legitimate risk for patients who *already have* kidney problems due to advanced diabetic complications. A higher-protein diet can potentially make it worse. But for those who have been recently diagnosed with diabetes or prediabetes, a diet built around protein-rich foods can ultimately *prevent* kidney damage by helping you lose weight, lower blood sugar, and improve insulin sensitivity.

The case for bone damage, on the other hand, is entirely speculative. The idea is that a diet higher in protein (as well as grains) creates a higher acid load in your blood, which in turn pulls calcium from bones, making them weaker. There's no evidence that dietary protein has any negative effect on bone health. In fact, stronger muscles—built with exercise and supported by protein—should make bones *stronger,* not weaker.

You might also hear that protein in general, and from red meat in particular, is linked to a higher risk of type 2 diabetes. This association comes from massive epidemiological studies involving many thousands of subjects followed for decades. When the researchers compared those who eat the most protein to those who eat the least, they found a 7 percent higher rate of diabetes among those who eat the most protein. For animal protein specifically, it was 13 percent, compared to a slightly lower diabetes risk for those who eat the most vegetable protein.

It's important to note that the studies aren't interventions in which scientists deliberately change someone's diet to see what happens. And they certainly aren't looking at a population that's focused on weight loss. One of the biggest challenges of studying the health effects of protein is that the people who eat the most are the least likely to exercise and the most likely to smoke and have obesity. In other words, in studies of large populations, the ones who eat the most protein typically eat the most, period.

As a result, researchers have to make statistical adjustments to account for those factors. The studies I just mentioned adjusted for age, weight, smoking, activity level, and family history of diabetes. In one analysis of their massive pool of data, researchers looked specifically at red meat and the associated risk of type 2 diabetes. They found that, compared to the people who ate the least red meat, those who ate the most were 14 percent more likely to have diabetes.

That's certainly good to know, but even more important is this finding: The diabetes risk for those who ate the most *processed* red meat—bacon, sausage, hot dogs, lunchmeat—was 32 percent higher. For each 50 grams of processed red meat per day, your risk for diabetes goes up by 51 percent. That's one hot dog (45 grams) and one slice of bacon (8 grams).

The risks are considerably lower for unprocessed red meats, like beef, pork, or lamb. If you eat 100 grams a day—roughly 3½ ounces, or a portion that's slightly larger than a bar of soap—your risk increases by 19 percent.

Interestingly, the same research shows a *lower* diabetes risk when meat eaters substitute a serving of nuts, whole grains, poultry, or low-fat dairy for a serving of red meat.

My advice is simple and easy to remember.

- ***Avoid processed red meats whenever possible,*** just as you avoid other highly processed foods. A slice of bacon with Sunday brunch, or some grilled bratwurst at a tailgate party, isn't going to kill you. But having bacon, sausage, or lunchmeats on a daily basis is a terrible idea.

- ***Enjoy red meat as a small part of your overall diet,*** just not every day. An occasional burger for lunch or pot roast for dinner easily fits into my idea of a healthy diet.

- ***Poultry, fish, dairy, and eggs are great sources of animal protein.*** Enjoy them as much as you want.

- ***Vegetable proteins are great choices, for multiple reasons.*** Legumes like beans and peas are high in fiber and moderately rich in protein. And because they're whole, unprocessed foods, they also have a wide range of vitamins and minerals. The same goes for whole grains, even though they're lower in both protein and fiber.

## CHAPTER 9

# Understanding Fat as Neither Friend nor Foe

**THERE WERE TIMES IN HUMAN HISTORY** when fat was hard to come by. Game animals were extremely lean, and when our ancient ancestors managed to kill one, they immediately ate the brain. It was the greatest source of fat, and also the most challenging to transport. Same with bone marrow. Because the bones of some of those animals were so heavy, they would sometimes crack them open and slurp down the marrow before carrying the meat back to their families. Hunters developed methods to get the fat from wherever animals stored it—organs, bones, tails, even testicles—and made a point of consuming every last globule. Their survival depended on it.

Fat fulfills multiple needs in our diets. Some fats are considered "essential" because we can't synthesize them from other types of nutrients, and without them our health would suffer. We need fat to absorb vitamins A, D, E, and K; to keep our skin and hair from drying out; to support our joints; and to keep our immune system up and running.

But mostly we need fat for energy, thanks to that amazing fuel-guzzling organ between our ears, which uses 20 percent of our daily calories—far more than the brains of other mammals our size. Prehistoric people ate brains to support brains. Because fat supplies the majority of the energy our bodies use over the course of the day, our appetites evolved over millions of years to give us what we need: a diet with the most concentrated nutrients, which means a hereditary preference for fat.

## WHAT IS FAT?

This question is more complicated than it seems. Fat is not all one thing. When we talk about fat, we're usually talking about *fatty acids*. Remember how I said protein is made up of 20 amino acids, arranged in different ways? Same with fat, except there are many times more arrangements. Milk fat, for example, includes 400 different fatty acids. All of them have different chemical structures and do slightly different things.

Most fats are bundled up into *triglycerides*—three fatty acids plus a "backbone" of glycerol. (Glycerol is a type of carbohydrate called a sugar alcohol, although technically it's neither sugar nor alcohol. Isn't biochemistry fun?) Most of the fat you eat, from animals or plants, is in the form of triglycerides. The triglycerides are broken up during digestion into fatty acids, just as protein is broken down into amino acids. Most of it then reforms into triglycerides before it enters your bloodstream.

Insulin comes into play, pushing some of those triglycerides into your fat cells, while others are used directly for energy. But when you're insulin resistant, a very odd thing happens: Free fatty acids stream out of your fat cells while triglycerides struggle to get in. Those fatty acids flow to your liver, where they're reconstituted into triglycerides.

Now we get to the part that's *really* complicated. Triglycerides can't get around your bloodstream by themselves. They need a vessel. That vessel is a *lipoprotein*. You've heard of the two major types: high-density lipoprotein (HDL), which is usually referred to as good cholesterol (although cholesterol itself is only a small part of the package, as I'll explain in a moment), and low-density lipoprotein (LDL), aka bad cholesterol.

Cholesterol is a substance that gives cells both structure and flexibility. Without structure your cells wouldn't exist, and without flexibility you wouldn't be able to move. Cholesterol is so important that every cell in your body can manufacture it. But some tissues need a little more, and lipoproteins make sure it gets there.

## THE PERILS OF A "HEALTHY" ROUTINE

Here's a problem I never anticipated when I started my career in medicine: How do I help patients unlearn outdated information? My older patients grew into adulthood at a time when everyone *knew* that eating fat made you fat, and everyone *knew* that eating food with cholesterol gave you heart disease. The less dietary fat and cholesterol you consumed, the healthier you'd be.

So they built their daily routines around high-carbohydrate, low-fat meals. A typical daily breakfast is a bowl of cereal, a muffin, and/or a glass of orange juice. It wouldn't be accurate to say that kind of diet *causes* type 2 diabetes, but once you have the disease, high-carbohydrate meals like the breakfast I just described undoubtedly make it worse.

At the same time, many of these patients are still afraid of fat and cholesterol. So that's two challenges for me. I have to persuade them to stop building every meal around carbohydrates, and also convince them it's okay to have ham and eggs for breakfast.

One trick that works for everyone who tries it:

I ask them to double the vegetables on their plate while cutting in half the portion of pasta, potatoes, or bread they would normally have. It works because they feel just as full while eating fewer calories. And without the spike in blood sugar that comes with a high-carb meal, they feel more energetic afterward, creating the perfect conditions for a post-meal walk.

Now that's a recipe for a healthy life!

What all fat has in common, when it's in the form of triglycerides, is that it provides 9 calories of energy per gram—more than twice what you get from carbs or protein. A typical American adult gets 33 percent of all calories from fat. That number has barely changed over recent years, despite concerted efforts by the government and health organizations to get us to eat less.

Dietary fat is usually classified as either saturated or unsaturated. Unsaturated fats are divided into monounsaturated and polyunsaturated, and then polyunsaturated fats are further divided into two major categories: omega-3 and omega-6 (the "essential" fats).

Got that?

It's okay if you don't. If I were trying to write a bestselling diet book, I'd pick one type of fat and convince you that eating more or less of it is the key to effortless weight loss. I might make a lot of money, but I doubt if I would help many people achieve their goals. Human metabolism is far too sophisticated for such minor tweaks to result in major changes to the size and shape of your body.

To be clear, some of these distinctions do matter when it comes to your health. I've seen both positive and negative changes to my patients' blood work that we could link to changes in dietary fat. But our focus in this book is to reverse diabetes and reduce obesity. For that, *the total amount of food you eat,* combined with physical activity, matters far more than which type of fat you ate slightly more or less of.

So why do we think these specifics matter so much more than they do? For that, let's take a short trip back in time.

## WHY WE'RE SO CONFUSED ABOUT FAT

Back in 1947, Ancel Keys was concerned about the epidemic of heart attacks. Why were so many apparently healthy men dropping dead? What was different about them? Keys at the time was one of the country's most respected scientists. He's the guy who developed K rations for our soldiers in World War II (the "K" is for Keys), and he also conducted what became known as the Minnesota starvation experiment, in which conscientious objectors to military service volunteered to lose and then regain 25 percent of their body weight. The goal was to gain knowledge that would save the lives of millions of civilians who'd been malnourished to the brink of death by the war. Now, in the postwar years, he set out to save millions who were dying of excess nutrition.

Keys was a few years into his research when he visited Italy and Spain in the early 1950s. There, he learned, men had much lower rates of heart disease, and he suspected it was because they ate so little meat and dairy. (Much of this early research focused

## THE CURIOUS CASE OF THE BUTTER IN THE COFFEE CUP

Nutrition fads come and go, and I'm as susceptible to them as anybody. Often they arise as a backlash against official guidelines that turn out to be misguided. That's how the relentless push to reduce fat fueled the popularity of low-carb diets. More recently, as we realized that saturated fats aren't as dangerous as we've been told, a handful of nutrition gurus have pushed them as *health* foods, telling their clients and fans to chow down on bacon, butter, whole milk, and fatty cuts of beef. This is pretty bizarre to me since those are all high-calorie foods, the last things I would recommend for patients struggling with obesity and diabetes.

Weirdest of all is a recent fad diet that recommends mixing butter and a special oil rich in medium-chain saturated fats into your coffee in the morning. Its biggest fans include bodybuilders and other extremely fit young men and women. But when I looked at the blood work of some of them, I hit the panic button. Their LDL cholesterol was sky-high. With typical patients, I would immediately prescribe statins to bring their cholesterol down and lower their risk of cardiovascular disease. But with these otherwise healthy individuals, I simply asked them to stop putting butter in their coffee. Their blood work improved dramatically.

entirely on men.) Those initial observations led to the Seven Countries Study, which, when published in 1970, cemented a national consensus around the idea that fat in general, and saturated fat especially, led to heart disease. The consensus had been building for a while. President Dwight Eisenhower, who'd suffered a heart attack in 1955, was convinced that saturated fat was responsible, and he took pains to avoid it. His cardiologist, Paul Dudley White, was a major proponent of the idea and had high praise for Ancel Keys and his work in establishing that link. The US government made it official policy to promote low-fat diets to prevent heart disease in 1977. And not just for those most at risk; this was the recommendation for *everybody* except infants and small children. The UK followed with its own call to reduce fat in 1983.

Unfortunately, the basic premise was wrong. A re-analysis of the data used to support those guidelines showed there was actually no difference in outcomes for those assigned low-fat diets. This makes sense when you consider how many different fatty acids there are, and how many different effects they have. Even the warnings about saturated fat may not have been warranted. Some researchers who've compiled and analyzed decades' worth of data now believe there's no link between saturated fat and either cardiovascular disease or premature death from any cause. Others still believe there is. Eisenhower himself was a cautionary example: He suffered six more heart attacks after he left office, despite his aversion to saturated fat.

And that brings me to the biggest point I'll make in this chapter: Your focus should be on whole foods that are rich in a variety of fats. Keep that in mind as we take a closer look at individual fats in the next section.

## MAJOR TYPES OF FAT

### Saturated Fat

**What it is:** The boilerplate description says you can identify saturated fats because they're solid at room temperature, like bacon grease or butter. But that's way too simple. Saturated fat shows up in meat, eggs, and dairy, where you expect it, but you'll also find small amounts in unexpected places, like vegetable oils, fish, nuts, and avocados. Nor is it helpful to think that saturated fatty acids are all the same. There are actually 36 different ones, each with its own name and functions. They're grouped into three categories—short-, medium-, and long-chain fatty acids—based on the number of carbon atoms.

**Benefits:** As it does with all fats, your body uses saturated fats for energy and will store them if you eat more than you need. They're also involved in hormone regulation and immune function, and they help provide structure to cells. But they're best known for raising cholesterol, and that's a concern if you already have cardiovascular disease or know you're at high risk. My basic advice to patients: Don't go out of your way to seek foods high in saturated fats, but don't avoid foods like meat, eggs, or dairy just because they have them.

## FOODS HIGH IN SATURATED FAT

| SOURCE | AMOUNT | TOTAL FAT (GRAMS) | SATURATED FAT (GRAMS) | OTHER BENEFITS/NOTES |
|---|---|---|---|---|
| Bacon | 1 slice | 3 | 1 | Like other meats, has protein, B vitamins, and minerals, but you really don't want to eat enough for those things to matter |
| Butter | 1 tablespoon | 11.5 | 7 | A little provides a lot of flavor and texture |
| Coconut oil | 1 tablespoon | 14 | 12 | Rich in medium-chain saturated fats |
| Dark chocolate | 2 ounces | 18 | 10 | Has a lot of sugar but is also packed with antioxidants |
| Egg | 1 | 6 | 2 | The fat-containing yolk is a third of the egg but contains most of the vitamins and minerals, and almost half the protein |
| Lean ground beef | 4 ounces | 23 | 9 | Great source of high-quality protein, B vitamins (especially $B_{12}$), and zinc |

# Monounsaturated Fat

**What it is:** I mentioned that the low rates of heart disease in Italy and Spain impressed Ancel Keys, who credited a lack of saturated fat. Researchers eventually noticed something else: The fat in the Italian and Spanish diets came largely from olive oil, a rich source of oleic acid, a monounsaturated fat (MUFA). But olive oil is just one of many foods with oleic acid. Meat and eggs are known for having a lot of saturated fat, but they actually have more monounsaturated. Salmon is justifiably touted as a great source of polyunsaturated fat, which I'll describe in a moment. But it too has more oleic. If you were a cannibal, you'd be happy to know that human fat is about 50 percent monounsaturated.

 **Benefits:** Olive oil has had incredible PR over the past few decades. Studies associate monounsaturated fats with lower risk of heart attacks and strokes, and modest

## FOODS HIGH IN MONOUNSATURATED FAT

| SOURCE | AMOUNT | TOTAL FAT (GRAMS) | MONOUNSATURATED FAT (GRAMS) | OTHER BENEFITS/NOTES |
|---|---|---|---|---|
| Almonds | ¼ cup | 15 | 9 | In long-term studies, people who eat the most nuts weigh less than those who eat the fewest |
| Avocado | ½ | 15 | 10 | Also has 5 grams of fiber |
| Canola oil | 1 tablespoon | 14 | 9 | Close to olive oil for monounsaturated fat |
| Cashews | ¼ cup | 13 | 7 | Decent source of protein and several minerals |
| Chicken breast | ½ | 13 | 5 | This is a bit of a cheat since I included the skin. I just wanted to show that you can get monounsaturated fat from almost any good protein source |
| Olive oil | 1 tablespoon | 14 | 10 | Extra-virgin is the best choice |
| Peanut butter | 1 tablespoon | 8 | 4 | Hard to stop at 1 tablespoon, which is the size of half a golf ball, making PB *way* too easy to overeat |

improvements in lots of other health measures. Most interesting, to me, is that foods high in these fats aren't linked with *any* negative effects on weight, blood sugar control, or cardiovascular risk. Even in studies that don't show clear benefits, we never see any risks. Does that mean olive oil is magic, and that you can slurp down as much as you want? I wouldn't go that far. But research consistently shows that when you substitute oleic acid for something else, your risk profile improves. When they're used as part of a healthy, calorie-controlled diet, you can't really go wrong with the foods shown in the chart opposite.

## Polyunsaturated Fat

**What they are:** Omega-3 and omega-6 polyunsaturated fats are "essential," which means your body can't make them from other fats. By contrast, you don't need to get any saturated fats from your diet, since your body can make them out of lots of things, including carbohydrates and alcohol. Polyunsaturated fats (PUFA) are almost always described as "good" or "healthy" fats. Sometimes they're combined in one category, and sometimes they're compared and contrasted. Omega-3 fats are found in relatively high amounts in nuts, seeds, fish, and fish oil. Omega-6 fats, on the other hand, have increased dramatically in the human diet, mostly from mass-produced oils added to processed food.

**What they do:** When researchers look at them separately, they've found that omega-3 fats are linked to lower risk of heart disease, less depression, and even better brain function. But it's unclear if you can get those benefits from fish oil supplements, or if you need to get your omega-3s from whole foods. For insulin sensitivity, omega-3 works well in rodent studies, but so far there's no compelling improvement for humans.

By contrast, omega-6 fats are kind of scary. Even though they're essential, this is the first time in human history when we've encountered these fatty acids in the quantities found in vegetable oils and processed foods. My recommendation: Don't worry about the omega-6 fats found in whole foods like fish, nuts, and seeds. But stay as far away as you can from the other stuff.

## FOODS HIGH IN POLYUNSATURATED FAT

| SOURCE | AMOUNT | TOTAL FAT (GRAMS) | POLYUNSATURATED FAT (GRAMS) | OTHER BENEFITS/NOTES |
|---|---|---|---|---|
| Fish oil | 5 grams | 5 | 2 | Best way to get omega-3, although benefits of supplements versus whole foods aren't clear |
| Flaxseeds | 1 tablespoon | 4 | 3 | Grind 'em up and sprinkle the powder over cereal or oatmeal, or add to a smoothie; you'll get 3 grams of fiber along with plant-based omega-3 |
| Salmon | 4 ounces | 14 | 5 | About half the polyunsaturated fat is omega-3 |
| Soybean oil | 1 tablespoon | 14 | 8 | Most of the omega-6 fats in modern diets come from soybean, corn, and cottonseed oils added to processed food |
| Walnuts | ¼ cup | 18 | 13 | Even with 2½ grams of omega-3, there is four times as much omega-6 |

## Trans Fats

To wrap up our discussion of fat, here's the one thing every nutrition expert agrees on: Trans fats are bad for you. Also referred to as partially hydrogenated fats, they're the unholy result of converting liquid vegetable oils into solid shortening or margarine for commercial food production. Chemically, hydrogenation makes the original polyunsaturated fats look more like saturated fats. But because they're human-made, the human body struggles to break them down. Trans fats cause damage to blood vessels and are linked to a scary-high risk of both type 2 diabetes and cardiovascular disease.

Americans have cut way back on trans fats since the 1990s, when we first learned how dangerous they are. By 2018 most will be banned altogether from commercial food manufacturing.

But that's not the whole story. Some trans fats occur naturally in ruminants—

animals that, succumbing to a level of boredom I can't even contemplate, spend all day rechewing and redigesting food they've already chewed and digested. You'll find small amounts of these natural trannies in cattle, sheep, and goats. About 2.7 percent of the fat in cow's milk is trans.

Conjugated linoleic acid (CLA) is the best known of these fats. All beef and milk products have some CLA; you'll find the most in full-fat dairy from grass-fed cows. Animal studies have shown that CLA reduces both body fat and cancer risk. This was great news for supplement manufacturers, who sold CLA as the latest and best fat burner. Human studies, alas, show modest fat reduction, if any at all. In my opinion they're a complete waste of money.

What can we learn from all this? Just what I've said a few times already: You'll get more from whole foods than their individual parts. Dairy offers a lot of health benefits to those who aren't lactose-intolerant. Some of those benefits come from dairy fat. Supplements can't compare.

So now that we've talked about weight loss in general, and taken more detailed looks at carbs, protein, and fat, it's time to put it all together into a sustainable diet plan.

# CHAPTER 10

# How to Build a Diet

**Way back in Chapter 3,** I said that I'm agnostic when it comes to diets. Low-fat, low-carb, paleo, vegan—all of them can help you lose weight and reverse diabetes. But the more extreme a diet is, the tougher it is to stick to it. The longer you go without eating foods that people normally enjoy, and that you've eaten for most of your life, the stronger your commitment to that diet needs to be. That's why the most ardent believers form cultlike communities around the nutrition plan they've chosen as the one true path to health and happiness . . . as you know if you've ever been stuck in a conversation with a militant follower of one of those diets.

The Mediterranean diet doesn't require a belief system, which is one reason I like it. It's also extremely flexible, as you'll see in a moment. There's no single version of the diet, no charismatic gurus promoting it, and no rival factions fighting over who has the purest interpretation of its principles. It's something you can talk about in polite company without much risk of a heated argument.

Among the benefits shown in research that compared the Mediterranean diet to a generic low-fat diet:

- Lower hemoglobin A1C

- More weight loss

- Higher HDL

- Lower rates of developing diabetes among those with the best adherence to the diet

But now I've used the word "diet" multiple times with the assumption that it means the same thing to all of us. So as I did in the previous chapters, I'll start by explaining what it means in this context.

## WHAT IS A DIET?

By definition, a diet is everything you eat on a regular basis. Which means everyone reading this has a diet. But the meaning changes when we put it into a sentence with a verb and a preposition. "I'm *on* a diet" or "I'm *going on* a diet" means you have changed or will soon change your habitual way of eating—for good reason, if you have obesity and/or diabetes.

Your instinct to change things up, perhaps drastically, is certainly well founded. When a team of researchers looked at every single hazard that ends life prematurely, or leads to disability, they found that dietary risks are the biggest danger in America today. "Composition of diet" accounts for 26 percent of deaths and 14 percent of "disability-adjusted life-years," which is a combination of years lost or severely compromised by a chronic condition. Smoking is a distant second.

Because the study was population-based and involved so much data I'd get a headache trying to imagine how they wrangled all of it, it doesn't go into many specifics about *why* American diets are so deadly. The major points—too few fruits and vegetables, too many trans fats and processed meats—are things you could easily guess after reading the previous chapters.

So when you think about "going on a diet," goal number one should be simple enough: Don't eat like a typical American. But that doesn't exactly narrow down your choices. Until someone invents the "Eat like a Numbskull and End Your Life Prematurely" diet, just about any plan you consider will clear that low hurdle.

Most will offer guidelines like these.

## What You *Should* Eat

A popular diet usually begins with a new or revived idea about which foods are the healthiest or best suited to specific goals like losing weight, building muscle, performing well in an endurance sport, or lowering your risk of heart disease or diabetes. Ideally, the one you choose will be based on foods you like and can continue to eat for the foreseeable future.

## What You *Shouldn't* Eat

Any good plan will probably tell you not to eat some of your favorite foods, especially the ones that are hard to stop eating once you start. The list will also include some "ah, screw it" foods, the things you eat only when you're too tired or rushed to prepare anything more appropriate to your goals. There might also be some you've simply eaten out of habit over the years without giving them much thought.

What this list *shouldn't* include are perfectly healthy foods that you're told to avoid for reasons you don't understand, or foods that are based on a fanciful imagining of what our ancestors ate before the devil invented agriculture, or on your blood type or the color of your hair or whether the food originated within some arbitrary radius of your neighborhood. (I just made up the one about hair color, but the others have all been popular in recent years.)

Unfortunately, it's *really* hard to tell the difference between solid and silly. A good marketer can make a ridiculous diet seem profound, with more study citations than a college textbook. But many of these diets are the scientific equivalent of a drunk in a bar explaining his favorite conspiracy theory.

- It starts with reasonable questions about something that invites skepticism.

- It segues to dark explanations of why we haven't yet found the answers, or how we settled on the wrong answers.

- And then it's off to crazy town.

I wish I had a clever way to detect the difference between good and bad science, but even scientists struggle with some of the big questions. All I can say with certainty is that I've never met a nutrition expert, in government or academia, who promotes a diet out of bad intentions. There are plenty of bad ideas and misguided policies, but I wouldn't call any of them conspiracies.

The combination of what you should and shouldn't eat will lead you, often indirectly, to . . .

## How *Much* You Should Eat

If a diet promises that you can eat all you want, never feel hungry, and still lose weight, I guarantee the diet will be so strict you have no choice but to eat less. And if you're eating less, at some point you're going to feel some hunger. The more ambitious you are, the more important it is to prepare for the inevitable. Some diets will give you specific calorie or macronutrient targets, which I'll talk about later in this chapter. The key point for now is that almost any structured plan will give you a way to eat less than you do now.

## *How* You Should Eat

A 19th-century fad diet created by Horace Fletcher required you to chew food 100 times per minute. His catchphrase: "Nature will castigate those who don't masticate." Other diet plans will specify a number of meals, or an amount of time between meals, or, in the case of fasting diets, that you don't eat anything at all for up to 24 hours at a time.

I'm no fan of Fletcherizing (that's what his fans called it), but the other instructions make sense, as you'll see in a moment. They aren't "rules" in the sense that you're doomed if you fail to follow them. But as guidelines, they give you structure to replace the randomness of free-range eating.

You can find lots of ways to impose your own rules or rituals on any eating plan. If you're somebody who eats over the stove, for example, you could set a place for yourself at the table, with a plate, napkin, silverware, and glass of water, and make it a rule that you can't take a bite unless you're seated at that place, with the food on the plate and the napkin on your lap. Another rule might be that you take a sip of water after every third or fourth bite.

Silly? Maybe. But if it works, who cares if it makes any sense?

# CLUB MED

And now we return to the Mediterranean diet. My modified version doesn't match up in all particulars with the diet used in research or promoted in popular cookbooks. But that's okay; those versions are essentially human creations, cherry-picked from what researchers thought were the healthiest choices in a region where people have lots of different eating patterns based on their culture, their proximity to the sea, their affluence or poverty, and what their land yields. In lieu of authenticity (I doubt if you'll find a single person living near the Mediterranean Sea whose diet matches what I'm about to describe), it meets my standards of a solid eating plan. That means it includes more protein than most people eat, and distributes that protein throughout the day.

Here it is in bullet points.

- Major sources of carbohydrates are fresh vegetables and fruits, legumes, and whole grains, more or less in that order, giving you a mix of sweet and filling foods with plenty of fiber.

- Major sources of fat include olive oil, nuts, fish, and/or cheese.

- Major sources of protein include fish, poultry, eggs, legumes, nuts, and cheese, with relatively little red meat, and as little processed meat as possible.

- If you need a snack, you'll want fruit and vegetables at the ready, with anything you're tempted to overeat kept out of sight and, ideally, out of mind.

- One or two alcoholic drinks after work and/or with dinner are acceptable, but by no means required.

- You'll try to avoid almost everything I discussed in Chapter 6, especially liquid calories from soda, juice, and flavored coffees and teas.

- Same with fast food, prepared dinners, and highly processed snacks and desserts—avoid, avoid, avoid.

- You don't need to be perfect, but you want to be consistent.

## MEAL FREQUENCY

I've seen diets that prescribed five or six feedings a day—three meals and two or three snacks—and others that called for a long daily fast, broken by one or two huge meals. I'm sure there are even more extreme ideas floating around. In the bodybuilding world, for example, people will obsess over what to eat before, after, and even *during* workouts. I've heard of young lifters being encouraged to wake up in the middle of the night for a snack, based on the absurd idea that they'll lose muscle if they go 8 hours without protein. But in my real-life practice, almost every patient eats three to four times a day. If that's your natural pattern, I see no reason to change it.

Within that pattern, however, my patients are all over the place. Some skip breakfast and have a light lunch, but also hit the vending machines every morning and afternoon. Some snack throughout the day, turning three square meals into one big amoeba-shaped feast.

So here are the first three guidelines.

1. Aim for the same number of meals every day.

2. Try to have those meals at the same times every day. You'll notice how this syncs up with the sleep habits I talked about in Chapter 5—get a consistent amount of sleep each night by going to bed and waking up at the same times.

3. Try to put at least 4 hours between each meal. It takes your body about 3 hours to process a normal-size meal. After that, your body relies more on stored fat and carbohydrate for energy. That easy flow of nutrients into and out of cells is a hallmark of a healthy metabolism.

## TOTAL CALORIES

I don't often recommend counting calories, especially for someone who's just starting out. The basic behavior- and environment-modifying techniques I described in Chapter 6 can be challenging enough on their own. And for those who embrace and master them, they might do the job of reducing total calories without making any other changes. Some patients don't even need the entire list; just taking a daily walk and cutting out liquid calories from soda, juice, and coffee can jump-start weight loss and bring blood sugar down.

But if you've already plucked that low-hanging fruit, or if you just like keeping track of things, a daily calorie target might be useful. There are two ways to do it.

- Count up the number of calories you actually eat, without attempting to change anything; calculate the average over 3 to 5 days; and then figure out how to reduce that number by several hundred a day.

- Estimate how many calories you *should* eat to reach a specific target weight, and figure out how to hit that target.

For the latter approach, you can find sophisticated calculators, apps, and wearable trackers that will estimate your metabolic rate and recommend a target. The one I recommend is the Body Weight Planner developed by the National Institute of Diabetes and Digestive and Kidney Disease (niddk.nih.gov/health-information/health-topics/weight-control/body-weight-planner/pages/bwp.aspx). It first asks you to enter your weight, height, gender, and age, and to estimate your activity level. You then input the weight you hope to achieve and when you hope to reach that weight, as well as how much additional exercise you're willing to do. Then it gives you three estimates.

- How much you probably eat now to maintain your current weight

- How much you need to eat to achieve your target weight by your target date

- How much you'll then need to eat to maintain that new, lower weight

I played around with the calculator, using some of my patients as examples, and it reminded me why I so rarely encourage them to count calories. If my most successful patients had looked at the numbers first, they might have given up before they even began. That's how daunting they are.

I'm also not sold on setting a target weight or a deadline to reach it. Most of us would pick an unrealistic weight and an even more unlikely time frame, and then feel like failures when we don't get close.

If you want to keep track despite those reservations, and think it will help you reach your goals, you still have the twin challenges of accountability and (rough) accuracy. The only way calorie counting works is if you count them all, which is harder than it sounds. The key steps:

- Measure and weigh everything you prepare at home, estimate the calories as closely as possible, and record the numbers in a journal or with an app. I recommend myfitnesspal.com, which is free and (relatively) easy to use.

- Look at the serving sizes on packages and be honest with yourself about how many servings you eat. This is especially important with sweets and desserts. The label on a carton of ice cream might say a serving is $\frac{1}{2}$ cup. But who in the world stops at a half cup? A typical dessert might be three servings. Same with a candy bar that says it's 200 calories per serving, and that there are $2\frac{1}{2}$ servings in a single bar. If you eat the whole thing, you have to count all 500 calories.

- When you eat at a chain restaurant, you might have to go online to find calorie counts for menu items. Even then, it's really just an estimate because a cook might use more butter or oil, or less of something else. This is why I recommend preparing your own food at home as often as possible.

- If there's no posted calorie count for one of your meals—lunch in a company cafeteria, say, or dinner at a non-chain restaurant—you have to estimate the serving size and then look up the calories. (I have specific tips in the next chapter.) You can easily find nutrition calculators online. They don't all agree with each other, but weight loss never hinges on a few under- or overestimated calories. It's the big stuff that matters. Just make sure you record *something* to account for everything you eat.

If these basic estimations are too far off, and you find yourself ravenously hungry because you've cut too much, or you aren't losing weight because you haven't cut enough, you can always make simple adjustments up or down. Keep in mind that your goal isn't to track calories into perpetuity (unless you like doing it). It's to quantify how much you eat *now* and to give you a baseline from which you can reduce calories.

## MACRONUTRIENTS

Quantifying macronutrients is one way to get around having to count every calorie. The Zone diet, for example, famously advocated a 40-30-30 ratio of carbs, protein, and fat. To mainstream experts in the mid 1990s, it was a shocking amount of protein and an equally shocking lack of carbohydrate. Even 30 percent fat was considered irresponsibly high at a time when those experts were gripped by low-fat mania. But the Zone diet was a huge and immediate hit with young athletes and fitness enthusiasts, and it stayed popular with them for a long time. (It was eventually eclipsed by the paleo diet.)

More recently, the acronym IIFYM—"if it fits your macros"—has become popular with that audience. The idea is to figure out what ratio of protein, carbs, and fat works best for your body and your goals, and then stick to it. Specific foods and eating behaviors are entirely at the discretion of the individual.

On the surface those plans sound simpler than calorie counting, but in practice they involve counting calories *and* counting grams of each macronutrient *and* calculating percentages.

A slightly less complicated practice is to quantify just one macronutrient. You can find lots of books that help you count grams of carbs, fat, and/or protein. If you're going to count anything, protein probably makes the most sense. Research shows that we eat less total food when 30 percent of our total calories come from protein. Eating 1 gram per pound of body weight will probably get you close to that target.

My recommendation, as you know from Chapter 8, is to aim for at least 30 grams of protein in at least three meals a day, including and especially at breakfast. We have solid research showing it reduces hunger, leading to less overall food consumed.

## SHOULD YOU AVOID CARBS?

In Chapter 7, I described the biggest problem with extremely restrictive diets: It's nearly impossible to stick with them. I know this from experience, having tried a super-low-carb ketogenic diet for a little more than a month. It "worked" in the sense that my blood sugar went lower. I ate less and eventually felt pretty good. But to make it work, I had to become a complete pain in the neck to my wife and friends. You can't even pretend to be a normal person with a normal life.

"Ketogenic" means your body is in a state of ketosis, which means there isn't enough carbohydrate to keep it running. Your body freely taps into its supply of stored fat, and supplements it with chemicals called ketone bodies. Those ketone bodies are produced primarily in your liver through a process too complicated to explain here. (If the word "acetyl-CoA" sounds interesting, you're free to Google it.) This is what matters: Every part of your body that runs on glucose, with the exception of red blood cells, can also run on ketone bodies.

You can put yourself into ketosis with a super-low-carb diet. That's roughly 20 to 50 grams a day (for reference, a medium banana has 25 grams), with carbs providing less than 10 percent of your total calories. Or you can do it by fasting

You also know from Chapter 7 that I recommend limiting carbohydrates to 40 net grams (total carbs minus fiber) per meal. That's mainly to help you control blood sugar, although I also think it's easier to eat less with lower-carb meals. But because carbs trigger the release of serotonin, a mood-stabilizing hormone (among many other roles), it's hard for many of us to feel satisfied without *some* carbs in the meal.

That leaves fat. Logic says it's not possible to eat a higher-protein, lower-carb diet that's also low in fat, unless it's super-low in calories, which isn't sustainable. So, by necessity, the sample meals you see in the next chapter may have more fat than you're used to. The key to making this plan (or, really, any plan) work is to put

or eating an extremely low-calorie diet. If you do, your blood sugar will drop, your insulin sensitivity will improve, and you will probably lose weight, although weight loss isn't necessary to get the other benefits.

A ketogenic diet can be lifesaving for someone with epilepsy whose seizures can't be controlled any other way. For type 2 diabetes, it can be a successful but extremely challenging intervention. I recommend it only to patients who have had the disease for a long time—usually a decade or more—and who are open to the idea. For example, if a patient tells me she used the low-carb Atkins diet successfully in the past and has no problem with the limited menu choices, I do what I can to help her make it work.

I have several patients who have used the diet successfully. It seems to work best when you join a supportive online community and make the diet part of your life. But it really does require that kind of long-term commitment. Adherence is everything. Once your doctor adjusts your medications to fit the new diet—without adjustment, there's a *serious* risk of hypoglycemia—you can't just decide one day that you're in the mood for a piece of pie.

together a combination of foods that allows you to eat the fewest calories without leaving you uncomfortably hungry between meals.

## "CHEAT" MEALS

Anyone following an extremely strict diet will, at some point, get fed up with not feeling filled up. Obesity specialists like me will say that it's okay to slip up. It's not that big of a deal. Just go right back to the program as if it never happened. But some in our audience don't hear it that way. To them, it's like an alcoholic falling off the wagon. Instead of being able to say, "My last chocolate-covered corn dog was 7 weeks ago," they're back to square one.

That's why some diets now encourage a regular cheat meal, or perhaps an entire day of unrestricted eating. In theory, it's easier to stick it out for 6 days if you know you can eat anything you want on the 7th. Then, having satisfied your pent-up cravings and eliminated your sense of deprivation, you get back to the diet the next day. In fact, a massive refeeding should make it even easier to restrict yourself, at least for the first day or two.

I get all that, and I've seen it work. But I still don't advocate cheat meals.

Your success in losing weight and defeating diabetes depends on self-management—being in control of your behavior and continually aware of how your behavior leads you closer to your goals. I don't like to encourage any behavior that takes you farther away.

Here's what can happen: Let's say you let yourself go on Sunday—pancakes, pizza, whatever your trigger is. But a couple days later, you actually weigh less than you did on Sunday morning. You think, "Hey, I found a loophole!" You try it again the following Sunday, and once again, you don't gain any weight from the episode. You start to think that maybe all the restrictions you imposed on yourself weren't necessary after all. While Sunday is still your designated "cheat" day, you give yourself permission to loosen things up on other days. Instead of pushing away from the table when you're satisfied, you eat until you're full. By the time the weight you lost has come back, you have abandoned the plan altogether and feel like a failure.

I prefer "normal person" meals.

Every now and then, when the opportunity arises, go out with family or friends and act like a normal person—not necessarily your old self, but someone who's not focused on weight loss. If you can limit these "normal person" meals to special occasions (and don't define "special" as "Thursday"; if it happens every week, it's not special), you accomplish the goals of a cheat meal without actually cheating. You're not washing down an extra-large pizza with a six-pack of Sam Adams. You aren't ordering three desserts and then turning to your companions and saying, "So what are you guys getting?" You're just eating a good, satisfying meal like everyone else in the room.

## MEAL REPLACEMENTS

Sometimes you're too rushed, stressed, or unmotivated to prepare any kind of meal, "normal" or otherwise. That's where meal-replacement smoothies come in. They have four crucial benefits.

- You can't beat the convenience of a meal that's ready in less than 5 minutes.

- There's no easier way to get 30 grams of protein, or any other specific amount.

- It's a great way to work in one or two servings of fruit.

- You know exactly what you're getting, and you can easily and simply account for everything in the smoothie—protein, calories, fiber, etc.

Remember the Look AHEAD study that I described in Chapter 3? The one that looked at long-term weight loss among people with diabetes? In the first year of the study, the plan relied heavily on meal replacements. The participants who used them the most—12 per week—lost 11.2 percent of their initial body weight, on average. Those who averaged just two per week lost 5.9 percent of their weight.

Satiety is a major reason why they work so well. Study subjects who get a drink made with whey protein are less hungry between meals, and subsequently eat less at the next meal. For those with diabetes, there's an added benefit: Whey slows down

# HIGH SATIETY

Back in 1995, researchers at the University of Sydney in Australia developed the satiety index, ranking 38 foods based on which ones offer the most satisfaction between meals. Here's a sampling. A number greater than 100 means the food is more satiating than white bread; less than 100 means it's less satiating.

| FOOD | SATIETY INDEX |
|------|---------------|
| Boiled potatoes | 323 |
| Oatmeal | 209 |
| Apple | 197 |
| Beef | 176 |
| Baked beans | 168 |
| Whole wheat bread | 157 |
| Eggs | 150 |
| Cheese | 146 |
| White rice | 138 |
| Lentils | 133 |
| Brown rice | 132 |
| Banana | 118 |
| White bread | 100 |
| Ice cream | 96 |
| Peanuts | 84 |
| Cake | 65 |

*Source:* SH Holt et al., "A satiety index of common foods." *European Journal of Clinical Nutrition* 1995; 49 (9): 675–90.

The higher-protein foods (beef, eggs, cheese, lentils) are a lot more satiating than white bread, as you'd expect. Whole wheat bread is 57 percent more satiating than white bread—again, no surprise. It's a little odd to see white rice ahead

the rate at which food hits your bloodstream, which means you get a smaller rise in blood sugar. At the same time, you get a larger increase in insulin, a boost that helps get nutrients out of your blood and into your cells, leading to lower A1C over time.

of brown, but they're so close it's hard to imagine you'd notice the difference.

But right at the top of the list, you see an obvious outlier: potatoes. You may remember from Chapter 7 that baked potatoes are at the top of the glycemic index, the measure of which carb-rich foods reach your bloodstream fastest. They also ranked near the top for glycemic load, which looks at the blood sugar response from a typical serving size instead of using 50 grams (just under 2 ounces) for everything.

One *possible* explanation is that potatoes provoke an extremely high insulin response, as do baked beans. And insulin, as problematic as it is for someone with diabetes, also has a powerful appetite-suppressing effect. It makes sense when you think about the sequence.

1. **You eat a meal with a lot of carbs.**

2. **Glucose hits your bloodstream.**

3. **Your pancreas releases insulin.**

4. **While insulin works to push glucose and fat into storage, it also shuts down your appetite, since more food would just make the job harder.**

It doesn't work that way with everything. Apples, for example, have a low glycemic index and load, a low insulin response, and a very high satiety effect. So how do you predict how satisfying a food will be, short of memorizing a list like this one? First, and most important, is to keep in mind that we rarely eat just one food at a time. (Apples, conveniently, might be an exception.) When you combine foods, you can't really go wrong with the principles I've described in this book: Focus on whole foods, with a bias toward those high in protein and fiber. Satiety will take care of itself.

I recommend a basic whey protein powder, which you can get just about anywhere these days—grocery stores, online, Costco or Sam's Club, or a dedicated supplement store like GNC. Choose one that's artificially sweetened, or at worst has a small amount of added sugar. Use enough to reach 30 to 40 grams of protein. You can simply blend it up with a few ice cubes, or you can make it a true meal by adding fruit, nut butter, and/or a flavored oil.

You can get even more out of a smoothie by making it as thick as possible. In a study that came out in 2016, a team of Dutch researchers showed that the "phantom fullness" created by a more viscous shake had a profound effect on satiety. Those who got shakes artificially thickened by a food additive were full longer (it took an additional 15 minutes for the first half of the shake to work through the digestive process) and had much lower hunger ratings and desire to eat.

The researchers used locust bean gum—a fiber extracted from carob—to create phantom fullness. I'm sure it's perfectly safe, but it's not something I've ever tried, and thus I can't recommend it. But there are a few easy ways to make your shake thicker, and thus more filling and satisfying.

Start with less water than the label or recipe suggests. If you're using multiple ingredients—fruit plus some kind of butter or oil—blend those up before adding ice. Then add ice (crushed, if you have it) and blend that in to reach your desired thickness.

Those are the basic rules and features of the diet program. You'll find specific meal ideas in the next chapter.

## CHAPTER 11

# Your Go-To Meals

**EVERY DIET FEELS STRANGE AT FIRST,** with unfamiliar food choices and lots of adjustments. That's why so few of them stick. They never stop feeling strange. But a good diet, a sustainable diet, doesn't *feel* like a diet. It doesn't seem unnatural or require constant monitoring and self-restraint. You don't wake up in the morning confused about what you can and can't eat that day. You just know.

So what makes a diet so familiar that it's automatic?

*Your go-to meals*—the breakfasts, lunches, dinners, and snacks that you can buy or throw together without much thought or planning.

Most of us tend to eat the same things out of habit and convenience. We're all busy, and none of us has the time or mental energy to plan and prepare new and interesting meals multiple times a day. Even when we grab lunch on the run or go to a favorite restaurant for dinner, we typically default to meals that we're familiar with and that we know will hit the spot. We know we'll get the volume and flavors we need to walk away both sated and satisfied. Ideally, we won't need to think about food again for the next few hours.

But here's the challenge for you.

When you are overweight and have diabetes, your go-to meals are part of the problem. They provide too many calories or too little satiety. Or maybe they're part of a pattern that reinforces other habits you'd like to break. Sweets for breakfast, for example, could trigger cravings for a midmorning vending-machine snack. A lunch that's too light could leave you ravenous long before dinner. A dinner that's too carb-heavy—or too heavy, period—could drain you of energy for the rest of the evening, so instead of a post-meal walk, you take root on the sofa, where you watch TV until bedtime. If you have a self-destructive habit you want to break, chances are it's entwined with a meal pattern that's dangerous to your health.

This chapter has two parts. First I'll review the nutrition parameters from the previous chapter, in order of importance (more or less). Then I'll show you how to apply them to some simple meal templates, including some suggestions for smoothies that you can use as meal replacements any time of day, and a list of some dishes you can order at popular chain restaurants that hit the targets. You'll find more (and more complex) recipes in Appendix A, and in Appendix B you'll see some suggestions for how to put the go-to meals together into daily meal plans for a variety of calorie levels.

## WHAT MATTERS MOST

Here's what you need your go-to meals to help you achieve.

1. Eat at least three meals a day, with at least 30 grams of protein in each one. That includes breakfast (or whatever you call your first meal of the day). Along with protein, you want to include highly satiating foods in each meal—whole grains, legumes, and fruits and vegetables.

2. Limit each meal to 40 grams of net carbs (total carbs minus fiber). For snacks, keep it to 20 grams (one medium apple) or fewer.

3. Include some fat in each meal. The best sources include olive oil (for cooking or in salad dressing), nuts, eggs, dairy, fish, meat, and avocados.

4. Aim for at least 4 hours between meals. Your goal is to be genuinely hungry for each meal, but not so ravenous that your hunger distracts you from whatever you're supposed to be doing.

5. Prepare as many meals as possible at home, including a lunch to bring to work, if that's practical for you.

6. Serve your meals using smaller plates, bowls, or glasses than you've traditionally used. The portions will look bigger, and you'll be no more tempted to go for seconds.

7. Drink a glass of water with each meal, or a calorie-free beverage like tea or coffee. It will stretch your stomach and allow you to feel full sooner.

8. A glass of wine with dinner or a beer or cocktail after work is fine. Two a day should be the limit for men; women will do best if they stop at one.

9. Once a week or so, preferably on a special occasion, enjoy a "normal person" meal. This isn't a "cheat" meal. You still want it to meet *most* of the imperatives on this list. But it's okay to eat something a little sweeter or creamier, or have a larger serving, or otherwise feel like you're indulging yourself a bit more than usual.

And here's what you'll try to avoid.

1. Most beverages with calories—sodas, flavored teas, juices, dessertlike coffees, or alcoholic drinks with any of those ingredients.

2. Carbohydrate-rich meals with minimal protein or fat. These include sandwiches that are mostly bread; pasta dishes that are mostly pasta; thick- or stuffed-crust pizza; and all-bread breakfasts—pancakes, waffles, French toast, etc.

3. Most prepared or packaged foods.

4. All deep-fried foods.

# GO-TO MEALS

The calorie counts for the following meals are taken from a variety of sources. Those sources often disagree with each other, which means they may also differ from the totals you see on a Web site or app. I also rounded up or down when necessary to keep the fractions under control. But the numbers should be close enough to give you an idea of how much you're eating.

Two important notes:

- You don't *have* to eat everything listed with a meal. Skip it if you don't think you need it.

- Feel free to add fruit or vegetables to any of these meals. Especially vegetables, which give you significant benefits with negligible calories.

# GO-TO BREAKFASTS

This is the meal most of us don't want to think about. If we eat breakfast at all, it tends to be the same thing every morning. So thinking about breakfast, and finding a way to get 30 grams of protein in your first meal each day, could be the biggest adjustment you make. But once you find a go-to combination of foods that works for you—one that tastes good, fills you up, and hits the protein target—breakfast should become as automatic as any other meal at any other time of day. If none of these is appealing, keep in mind that a breakfast smoothie, with 30 grams of protein from a supplement, is always an option.

# COTTAGE CHEESE WITH FRUIT AND NUTS

**FOR 1 SERVING:**

1 cup cottage cheese

¼ cup chopped walnuts

1 cup fresh fruit

*Totals: 477 calories, 33 grams protein, 14 net grams carbs (24 grams carbs, 10 grams fiber), 29 grams fat. If you use 1% fat cottage cheese, you can save 70 calories and 8 grams of fat.*

# HIGH-PROTEIN OATMEAL WITH CHIA SEEDS

**FOR 1 SERVING:**

1 cup cooked oatmeal

20 grams vanilla protein powder*

1 tablespoon chia seeds

*Totals: 316 calories, 28 grams protein, 29 net grams carbs (38 grams carbs, 9 grams fiber), 8.5 grams fat*

*\*This may be one scoop of your favorite brand, or it could be more or less. Different brands have different size scoops, and sometimes include carbs, fat, and/or fiber. For this example, I counted only 80 calories from 20 grams of protein.*

# NO-BRAINER EGGS

**FOR 1 SERVING:**

3 eggs, any style

2 ounces ham

1 slice whole wheat toast

1 orange

*Totals: 410 calories, 31 grams protein, 25 net grams carbs (30 grams carbs, 5 grams fiber), 24 grams fat*

# CHEESE AND VEGGIE OMELET

FOR 1 SERVING:

3 eggs

1 ounce part-skim mozzarella cheese

1 cup veggies (some combination of onions, tomato, mushrooms, bell peppers, spinach, etc.)

2 slices whole wheat toast

*Totals: 475 calories, 31 grams protein, 25 net grams carbs (30 grams carbs, 5 grams fiber), 23.5 grams fat. Substituting Cheddar, provolone, feta, or any other cheese will add or subtract a few calories. Same with the vegetables.*

# BREAKFAST BURRITO

FOR 1 SERVING:

2 eggs

½ cup chopped ham

¼ cup shredded Cheddar cheese

1 tomato, chopped

¼ cup chopped onion

1 tablespoon chopped cilantro

1 whole wheat tortilla (8" diameter)

*Totals: 444 calories, 34 grams protein, 27 net grams carbs (31 grams carbs, 4 grams fiber), 24 grams fat*

# CRABBY EGGS

FOR 1 SERVING:

3 eggs

2 ounces lump crab

½ cup cherry tomatoes, quartered

1 slice whole grain toast

Scramble the eggs with the crab and tomatoes, and serve on the slice of toast.

*Totals: 382 calories, 31 grams protein, 15 net grams carbs (18 grams carbs, 3 grams fiber), 19 grams fat*

*Recipe courtesy of Keri Glassman*

# GO-TO LUNCHES

The easiest lunch is leftovers from the previous night's dinner. Since you or your spouse prepared it, you know exactly what you're getting. When that's not an option, here are a few ideas for simple lunches you can prepare in a hurry.

## TURKEY SANDWICH WITH AVOCADO

FOR 1 SERVING:

3½ ounces turkey breast

2 slices whole wheat bread

½ cup sliced avocado

*Totals: 395 calories, 36 grams protein, 20 net grams carbs (29 grams carbs, 9 grams fiber), 14 grams fat*

**Note:** Avocados are a great source of monounsaturated fat, but they're pretty tough to account for when it comes to nutrition. The amount I chose is about ³⁄₈ of a standard avocado, which may be more or less than you'd actually use on a sandwich. It also leaves you with ⁵⁄₈ of an avocado to use in another meal.

## BIG SALAD

*I'll be honest: This is how I get rid of all the odds and ends I have left over from other meals. On any given day it includes some combination of meat, cheese, hard-cooked eggs, fruit, vegetables, and, of course, lettuce. So the following is just one possible version, which may have too much "big" and not enough "salad" for your taste.*

FOR 1 SERVING:

2 hard-cooked eggs

2 ounces chicken breast

2 cups chopped romaine lettuce

½ avocado

2 tablespoons balsamic vinaigrette

*Totals: 512 calories, 33 grams protein, 4 net grams carbs (13 grams carbs, 9 grams fiber), 41.5 grams fat*

# THE SANDWICH MATRIX

I don't know who first came up with the idea of putting meat or cheese or vegetables between two pieces of bread. I would guess it happened soon after some ingenious person thought to slice bread, instead of tearing it apart with fingers or teeth. It's generally acknowledged that the sandwich as we know it today was invented in 1762 by a cook working for the Earl of Sandwich, who demanded a meal he could eat without stepping away from whatever he was gambling on at the time.

Sandwiches have been part of everyday life in the United States for a couple hundred years. Which means they've probably been part of *your* life for as long as you can remember. Which also means they're part of the problem I described at the beginning of this chapter. If you are overweight and have type 2 diabetes, your regular eating habits—including those sandwiches—are almost certainly part of the problem.

I'm not saying you have to give up sandwiches; I included one in my suggestions for go-to lunches. You just have to use them intelligently. If you're not afraid

---

Low- or no-calorie components you can add for flavor and/or texture:

- Arugula
- Balsamic vinegar
- Cucumber
- Lettuce
- Mustard
- Onions
- Oregano
- Pepper, black
- Peppers
- Pickles
- Salt*
- Spinach
- Tomato

*There's no good reason to fear salt, unless you have hypertension and your doctor told you to cut back. Most of the sodium in our diets comes from the fast and prepared foods that you want to avoid anyway.

of a little math, the chart below shows how to put one together while getting at least 30 grams of protein and no more than 40 grams of net carbs. The usual caveats apply to the numbers for calories and grams of protein, carbs, fiber, and fat. We're *really* ballparking it here.

| COMPONENT | CALORIES | PROTEIN (GRAMS) | NET CARBS (GRAMS) | TOTAL CARBS (GRAMS) | FIBER (GRAMS) | FAT (GRAMS) |
|---|---|---|---|---|---|---|
| 2 slices of bread (whole wheat, rye, or pumpernickel) | 140 | 5 | 18 | 22 | 4 | 2 |
| 1 to 1¼ ounce cheese (1 slice Cheddar or Swiss, or 2 sticks string cheese, or 1¼ ounces mozzarella) | 100 | 7 | | | | 8 |
| 3 ounces deli turkey breast, roast beef, ham, or chicken (look for "no preservatives" on the package) | 110 | 25 | | | | 1 |
| ¼ avocado | 80 | 1 | 1 | 3.5 | 2.5 | 8 |
| 1 teaspoon olive oil | 40 | | | | | 4.5 |
| 1 tablespoon mayonnaise | 90 | | | | | 10 |

# TOTALLY NOT FROM THE MEDITERRANEAN BURRITO BOWL

*Like the Big Salad (on page 123), anything labeled as a "bowl" can be a great place to combine your orphaned ingredients. This bowl is itself an orphan: Even though the components are consistent with a Mediterranean-type diet, they come from all over the world. Black beans and tomatoes (in the salsa) originated in Central and South America; rice in China; cheese in the Mediterranean (among other places); and chicken, most likely, in Southeast Asia. If you want to tip the balance in favor of the Western Hemisphere, throw in some of that leftover avocado, which originated in Mexico.*

FOR 1 SERVING:

3 ounces chicken breast

½ cup black beans

1 ounce Mexican cheese blend

½ cup cooked brown rice

3 tablespoons salsa

*Totals: 455 calories, 43.5 grams protein, 38.5 net grams carbs (48 grams carbs, 9.5 grams fiber), 9 grams fat*

# GREEK TUNA SALAD

*The "Greek" part comes from artichokes (probably native to North Africa but used extensively in ancient Greece and Rome); feta cheese, made from the milk of sheep or goats; and arugula, a plant native to the region. According to Wikipedia, arugula was once considered an aphrodisiac, and thus forbidden in medieval monasteries (a story too good to bother verifying). Canned tuna isn't especially Mediterranean, but it's a great source of protein.*

FOR 2 SERVINGS:

1 can (5 ounces) light tuna in water

1 cup navy beans

1 can (14 ounces) quartered artichoke hearts

½ cup chopped cucumber

1 plum tomato

3 tablespoons olive oil

4 cups arugula

¼ cup crumbled feta cheese

Combine the tuna, beans, artichoke hearts, cucumber, tomato, and oil in a bowl, and toss it all together. Divide the arugula onto 2 plates. Scoop half the tuna mixture on each, with the feta on top. (Or save half for a future meal.)

*Totals (per serving): 488 calories, 33.5 grams protein, 13.5 net grams carbs (21.5 grams carbs, 8 grams fiber), 24.5 grams fat*

# CAPRESE SALAD

*Feeling lazy? Lunch doesn't get much easier (or more Mediterranean) than this.*

FOR 1 SERVING:

4 ounces part-skim mozzarella cheese, cut into ¼" slices

1 tomato, sliced

2 teaspoons extra-virgin olive oil

Fresh basil leaves

*Totals: 390 calories, 29 grams protein, 7.5 net grams carbs (9 grams carbs, 1.5 grams fiber), 27 grams fat*

# GO-TO DINNERS

If you're going to put a lot of thought into a meal, this is the one. Even your go-to dinners will probably take a bit more effort than the others. The following templates can be as simple as I describe, or as tasty and expertly prepared as you choose to make them. The ones described as a single serving can easily be scaled up to feed as many as you want. Be sure to factor leftovers into your dinner plans; as I said, last night's dinner is often the perfect lunch.

# STEAK, HOLD THE POTATOES

FOR 1 SERVING:

2 tomatoes, chopped

1 cucumber, peeled and chopped

1 onion, chopped

1 tablespoon lemon juice

6 ounces sirloin steak, grilled or broiled

2 cups broccoli, steamed

To make the cucumber salad, throw the tomatoes, cucumber, and onion into a bowl with the lemon juice. Add a bit of salt and pepper, stir, and either chill or serve at room temperature. Either way, it should make 2 servings. Grill or broil the steak while you steam the broccoli.

*Totals: 522 calories, 37 grams protein, 9 net grams carbs (16 grams carbs, 7 grams fiber), 34 grams fat*

# Super-Simple Slow-Cooked Chicken Chili

**FOR 8 SERVINGS:**

2 cans (15½ ounces each) kidney beans (dark, light, or one of each), rinsed and drained

1 can (15 ounces) tomato sauce

1½ cups salsa

2 tablespoons chili powder

3 pounds boneless, skinless chicken breasts, cut into small chunks

1 cup frozen corn

1 onion, chopped

1 ounce shredded Mexican cheese blend

Throw the rinsed beans, tomato sauce, salsa, and chili powder into a slow cooker and stir them up. Put the chicken, corn, and onion on top, but don't stir them until the chili is about halfway cooked. Cook for 6 to 8 hours on the low setting or about 4 hours on high. Serve with the cheese. Freeze whatever you won't consume for dinner or lunch in the next couple of days.

*Totals (per 1-cup serving): 508 calories, 68 grams protein, 24 net grams carbs (31 grams carbs, 7 grams fiber), 11 grams fat*

## Your Go-To Side Salad

*Feel free to add a salad to any lunch or dinner.*

**FOR 1 SERVING:**

2 cups mixed salad greens

1 cup cherry tomatoes (or any fruits or vegetables you prefer)

2 tablespoons balsamic vinaigrette

*Totals: 187 calories, 2 grams protein, 6 net grams carbs (10 grams carbs, 4 grams fiber), 16 grams fat*

# ROAST CHICKEN WITH SWEET POTATOES AND RED WINE

*I have to be honest: The calories and macronutrients I list for a dish like this are no better than a guess. Nutrition databases don't account for the supersize chicken parts you find in stores these days. There's also no precise way to estimate the vegetables you'll have in each serving, or how much of the fat from the chicken you'll consume (with leftovers, the fat will congeal on top, and you'll probably throw it out), or how much of the wine and tomato paste will evaporate while cooking, or how much wine you'll drink with dinner. (You'll have about 17 ounces left after you put 8 ounces—1 cup—on the chicken. A standard serving is 5 ounces.)*

*All that's in addition to the problems I mentioned at the beginning of the chapter: Different databases disagree on calorie counts, and even after I pick one, I still round up and down to avoid using fractions.*

*Calories aside, there's one sure way to eat a little less: Chew slowly and savor each bite, giving your stomach time to register the volume of food and drink and help you stop when you've had enough.*

**FOR 4 SERVINGS:**

- 1 cup red wine
- ¼ cup red wine vinegar
- ¼ cup tomato paste
- 2–3 sprigs fresh thyme
- ½ teaspoon dried oregano
- 4 chicken thighs
- 4 chicken drumsticks
- 2 sweet potatoes, chopped into bite-size pieces
- 6 carrots, cut however you like them
- 3 onions, cut into chunks

In a medium bowl, combine the red wine, vinegar, tomato paste, and herbs. Place the chicken in a shallow dish or resealable plastic bag and pour the wine mixture over it. Marinate in the refrigerator for 30 minutes or so while you prep the rest of the meal and preheat the oven to 400°F. Once the vegetables are cut, spread them across the bottom of a glass baking dish, and sprinkle a little water over them. Put the chicken on top of the vegetables and pour the marinade on top. Cover with foil and roast for 30 minutes. Take off the foil and roast for another 30 minutes, or until the chicken reaches 170°F, basting every 10 to 15 minutes.

*Totals (1 thigh and 1 drumstick per serving): 432 calories, 33 grams protein, 23 net grams carbs (28 grams carbs, 5 grams fiber), 21 grams fat*

# BAKED SALMON WITH GREEN BEANS

FOR 1 SERVING:

Pinch of dried dill

Pinch of dried basil

1 salmon fillet (6 ounces)

1 cup green beans

1½ cups chopped papaya

OPTIONAL:

1 teaspoon honey

1 teaspoon Dijon or stone-ground mustard

1 teaspoon lemon juice

1 tablespoon pistachios, chopped

To keep it really simple, rub some dried dill and basil onto the salmon, and bake at 375°F for 20 minutes or so. While it's baking, steam the green beans. Serve the cooked salmon with the papaya and green beans. For a heartier meal, top the salmon with a paste made with the honey, mustard, lemon juice, and pistachios, and bake as described. This one is easy to scale up for as many servings as you want.

*Totals (simple): 424 calories, 46 grams protein, 20 net grams carbs (27 grams carbs, 7 grams fiber), 14 grams fat*

*Totals (with pistachio mixture): 528 calories, 49 grams protein, 28 net grams carbs (36 grams carbs, 8 grams fiber), 20.5 grams fat*

# GO-TO SMOOTHIES

Smoothies are to contemporary diets what the Colt revolver (allegedly) was to the Wild West: a great equalizer. Those without time or culinary skills can throw together a meal replacement that's tasty and filling, and that hits all the benchmarks of a well-thought-out nutrition plan. You can reliably get 30 grams of protein with relatively few carbs. With a bit of planning, you can find ways to include nutrients that might otherwise go missing from your diet. It's easy to add fruit, fibrous vegetables, and a variety of fats from nut butters and oils.

The following is just a taste of the many ways you can replace an entire meal in just a few minutes with a handful of ingredients thrown into a blender. You'll probably need a few tries to get the flavors and texture to your liking. For example, you may prefer fresh fruit with a few ice cubes, rather than the frozen fruit I include in my recipes. But once your diet plan and tastebuds are on the same page, you can enjoy your go-to smoothie every day for years on end.

Final note: My calorie and macronutrient totals account for only the protein in the powder. If your supplement has added carbs or fat, adjust accordingly.

## THE STARTER KIT

*Here's the simplest base for a smoothie: your choice of protein powder (vanilla or chocolate), your choice of fruit, your choice of nut butter. You can skip the nut butter and throw in some actual nuts to make it crunchier, or use both to make it more filling.*

FOR 1 SERVING:

30 grams vanilla or chocolate protein powder

1 cup frozen raspberries

1 tablespoon cashew butter

8 ounces water

*Totals: 278 calories, 34 grams protein, 11 net grams carbs (19 grams carbs, 8 grams fiber), 8 grams fat*

# Every Day's a Holiday

*When I asked folks on Facebook to share their favorite smoothies, I got some amazing suggestions, most of which were too complicated, quirky, or caloric to include here. One persistent theme, though, was the creative use of flavorings like pumpkin pie spice, cinnamon, and nutmeg. This example comes from Will Katz, a fitness trainer in Kansas City, who says he's used it as his breakfast "virtually every day for years." I tweaked it a bit to reduce the carbs, but I left in the spinach, which he calls "free green stuff" because you get the vitamins and minerals without the otherwise strong taste. (I say that as someone who likes spinach but would never think to mix it with 2 spices I associate with Christmas.)*

**FOR 1 SERVING:**

20 grams chocolate protein powder

1 banana

½ cup frozen blueberries

2 whole eggs

Handful of baby spinach leaves

Dash of ground cinnamon

Dash of ground nutmeg

6–8 ounces water

*Totals: 385 calories, 32 grams protein, 34 net grams carbs (39 grams carbs, 5 grams fiber), 11 grams fat*

# The Breakfast Date

*I'd never heard of a Medjool date before a friend offered this recipe. To me, it sounds like a 3-year-old trying to say "medical school" (or me after a shot of Novocain). She recommended 2 to 4 dates per shake and raves about their sweet flavor, but since each date has 18 grams of carbs, I reduced it to 1. Feel free to increase the oatmeal for a crunchier texture, or to use dairy milk instead of almond. (Although if you go with dairy milk, I recommend using an unflavored protein powder.)*

**FOR 1 SERVING:**

20 grams plain or vanilla protein powder

1 Medjool date

1 tablespoon peanut butter

2 tablespoons rolled or steel-cut oats (raw, not cooked)

1 cup almond milk

*Totals: 408 calories, 28 grams protein, 36 net grams carbs (42 grams carbs, 6 grams fiber), 16 grams fat*

# Afternoon Delight

*The friend who recommends this one describes it as "Black Forest cake in a glass." I'll take her word for it. (I don't actually know what Black Forest cake tastes like, but it sounds good.) You can regard it as another building-block smoothie: Add a little nut butter to make it more substantial, use nonfat yogurt to cut the calories, or try your own combinations of fruit.*

FOR 1 SERVING:

20 grams chocolate protein powder

⅔ cup plain Greek yogurt

1 cup frozen cherries

1 cup almond milk

*Totals: 357 calories, 33 grams protein, 32 net grams carbs (35 grams carbs, 3 grams fiber), 10 grams fat*

## Don't Want to Drink Your Meal? Try a Smoothie Bowl

*When I called on my friends for shake ideas, I got this hybrid suggestion—a peanut, raspberry, and oats smoothie bowl—from nutritionist Elizabeth Ward, RD. It has a lot of ingredients, as you'll see, but protein powder isn't among them.*

FOR 1 SERVING:

½ cup fat-free plain Greek yogurt

¼ cup 1% milk

¼ cup peanut powder*

¼ cup uncooked oats

½ teaspoon vanilla extract

TOPPINGS

½ cup fresh raspberries

2 tablespoons chopped peanuts

Throw the yogurt, milk, peanut powder, oats, and vanilla in a blender or food processor. Blend on high speed until smooth. Pour into a cereal bowl, and put the raspberries and peanuts on top.

*Totals: 339 calories, 30 grams protein, 21 net grams carbs (31 grams carbs, 10 grams fiber), 7 grams fat*

*\*You'll find peanut powder in the aisle with nut butters.*

# GO-TO SNACKS

In a perfect world, one where you have control over when, where, and what you eat every single day, you could excise "snack" from your vocabulary. Each eating opportunity would be an actual meal that's at least 4 hours removed from the last one and 4 hours before the next. Control your nutrition and you control your blood sugar. Control your blood sugar and you control your health. You can see why I find the idea appealing.

But, alas, real life is many miles from perfect. Let's say you have lunch at noon, but dinner isn't until 7:00 or 8:00. And let's say you've learned the hard way that a heavy lunch leads to a sleepy, unproductive afternoon. So you're going to be hungry by 4:00 or 5:00 p.m., and you'll need something to hold you over until dinner.

Anything I've described so far in the breakfast, lunch, or smoothie categories could also make a fine snack. All of them can easily be whittled down to fit your immediate need. You don't have to worry about any particular amount of protein if you're getting at least 30 grams in three meals that day. You just need to make sure the snack hits the spot, within the parameters of this diet plan. Overshoot and you end up with more total calories than you need. Undershoot and you'll be hungry again before the next meal.

The perfect snack has *some* protein, although it doesn't need a lot. Fat will probably help in two ways—it'll feel more substantial and reduce any immediate cravings for carbs. And as always, you never want carbs to provide the bulk of the calories, even in a snack.

The chart on the next page lists a few foods you can combine in any way that appeals to you. You can pick up most of them on the fly; the rest you can have on hand for days when you might need them.

| FOOD | CALORIES | PROTEIN (GRAMS) | CARBS (GRAMS) | FAT (GRAMS) | FIBER (GRAMS) |
|---|---|---|---|---|---|
| 1 apple | 81 | | 21 | | 4 |
| ¼ cup (small handful) cashews | 155 | 5 | 9 | 12 | 1 |
| 1 cup cottage cheese | 232 | 28 | 6 | 10 | |
| 1 cup 0% Greek yogurt | 120 | 20 | 9 | | |
| 2 ounces part-skim mozzarella cheese | 144 | 14 | 2 | 9 | |
| 1 orange | 86 | 2 | 21 | | 4 |
| 2 tablespoons peanut butter | 188 | 8 | 6 | 16 | |
| ¼ cup (small handful) walnuts | 185 | 4 | 4 | 18 | |
| 1 slice whole wheat toast | 70 | 2.5 | 11 | 1 | 2 |

A few combinations:

- Peanut butter on apple slices or celery

- Fruit or nuts mixed into cottage cheese or yogurt

- Mozzarella cheese melted onto a thin slice of whole wheat toast

## GO-TO RESTAURANT MEALS

One thing that's changed a lot in the past few years: More chain restaurants now offer choices that meet all the criteria I've described for a healthy meal, with lots of protein, moderate fat and carbs, some fiber, and a reasonable amount of calories. The cost is more than fast food but a lot less than a high-end restaurant. In some places it isn't substantially more than you'd pay to buy and prep the food in your own kitchen, and the restaurant meal probably tastes somewhat better as well, depending on how you rate your own culinary skill.

The following are just a handful of options, based on restaurants I've been to or that my patients have mentioned. I didn't include a couple of popular ones either because I couldn't find good options or the nutrition data was incomplete. Cheesecake Factory, for example, had "n/a" in its protein column for every dish. Sorry, but protein is *extremely* "a" in a good diet.

| CHAIN | DISH | CALORIES | PROTEIN (GRAMS) | CARBS (GRAMS) | FAT (GRAMS) | FIBER (GRAMS) |
|---|---|---|---|---|---|---|
| Carrabba's | Shrimp & Sea Scallop Spiedino (skewer) | 550 | 38 | 11 | 38 | 1 |
| Chevy's Fresh Mex | Chicken Quesadilla (½ order; take the other ½ to go) | 540 | 26 | 39 | 31 | 1 |
| Chili's | Original BBQ Baby Back Ribs (half-rack) | 470 | 38 | 17 | 28 | 2 |
| Chipotle | Burrito Bowl (with chicken, black beans, salsa, cheese, guacamole) | 655 | 47 | 32 | 37 | 19 |
| Olive Garden | Garlic Rosemary Chicken* | 540 | 66 | 29 | 19 | 4 |
| Perkins | Mediterranean Omelet (no hollandaise sauce) | 445 | 26 | 17 | 30 | 4 |
| Red Lobster | Broiled Flounder Dinner (with asparagus and garden salad) | 630 | 78 | 35 | 18 | 7 |
| Red Robin | Ensenada Chicken Platter (2 chicken breasts) | 345 | 44 | 13 | 14 | 1 |
| Ruby Tuesday | Grilled Salmon (with sides of broccoli and zucchini) | 424 | 43 | 11 | 22 | 4 |
| Subway | Chicken Caesar Melt (6")** | 540 | 37 | 46 | 24 | 5 |

*There's a smaller version (400 calories) on the lunch menu.

**With 41 net carbs, it slips over my recommended limit. Leave a bit of the bread on your plate and you're good.

# ESTIMATING PORTION SIZES

If you're going to focus on calories, or protein grams, you need to measure portions as precisely as you can, as often as you can. In addition to the measuring cups and spoons you already have, I recommend getting an inexpensive food scale. I make good use of mine. (If I'm dieting for a specific goal, I might even bring it with me when I travel.) But no matter how precise you are, there will always be times when you need to estimate the size of a portion with nothing but your eyeballs. These are some easy guidelines.

**Meat or fish.** It's customary in a diet book to say that 3 ounces is the size of a deck of cards or bar of soap. But when's the last time you saw a portion that small? A more realistic cut like 6 ounces should be about the size and thickness of your palm and fingers (unless you have unusually big or small hands), or two checkbooks.

**Semisolid food.** A tablespoon of butter is the size of the top half of your thumb (from the last knuckle to the tip). Two tablespoons of peanut butter is proportional to a golf ball. A half-cup of ice cream is about the size of a tennis ball. Or, if you can't picture it fully rounded, imagine a small apple cut in half. Each piece would be a half-cup.

**Cheese.** If you can picture it cubed, 1 ounce would be four dice, or the size of your entire thumb. If it's flat, imagine three dominoes.

**Nuts and seeds.** The standard portion can be expressed three different ways: 28 grams, 1 ounce, or slightly less than ¼ cup. With your palm cupped, it should just fit without spilling over.

**Fruits and vegetables.** A cup is about the size of a man's fist, whether it's raspberries or salad greens.

**Rice.** A cupcake wrapper filled with rice would be a half-cup. So a cup would be like two homemade cupcakes with the tops cut off.

# PART THREE

# TRAIN TO GAIN

## CHAPTER 12

# How to Begin
# a Fitness Program

**PART TWO FOCUSED** on what you lose by modifying your diet: weight, fat, high blood sugar. Now it's time to focus on what you gain from fitness. Most of this chapter, by necessity, focuses on strength training, where the goal is to build strength and increase the size of your muscles. I say that knowing the idea of gaining *anything* is upsetting to many of my female patients, especially the ones who grew up in a world where a woman simply did not pick up a heavy thing unless one of her children was trapped beneath it. If you spent 75 percent of your life under the assumption that the thinnest person is the most appealing and valued, why would you set out to make your body bigger?

Rest assured "bigger" isn't the objective. We're shooting for "better." Leaner. Lighter. Stronger. More energy. Better endurance. Quicker strides. Improved balance and mobility. Less joint pain. More self-confidence and a powerful sense of accomplishment. You can gain all that and more with the relatively simple exercise program I'm about to prescribe.

# PART ONE: THE FIRST STEP(S)

This is as close as I can get to providing white-coat, stethoscope-around-my-neck medical advice to someone I haven't examined: *I expect every ambulatory person reading this book to walk for at least 30 minutes a day.*

It's the bare minimum, and you can't allow yourself to make excuses for not doing it. It's dark outside? Take a flashlight and wear a reflective vest. Cold? Put on thermal underwear, two pairs of socks, and as many sweaters and jackets as you need. Hot? Protect your skin and bring a water bottle.

And if 30 minutes a day isn't enough? Now we're talking my language. Here's how to make progress.

**Increase the frequency.** Aim for a short walk after every meal. Or, if that's not practical, at least get up and stretch your legs, move your arms, straighten your back, and reset your shoulders every half-hour or so.

**Increase the duration.** When 30 minutes is a cinch, increase your daily walk—or your longest walk of the day—to 45 minutes, then 60. From time to time, when your schedule allows, go even longer. And if you get the opportunity, go *really* long by hitting a trail and taking a hike.

By increasing your endurance, you improve the function of your heart and lungs. More oxygen gets into your blood, it circulates farther, and it gets there faster. More glucose and fat enter and leave your bloodstream. Even your brain function improves. Over time, endurance exercise has powerful mood-altering effects, simultaneously acting as a stimulant, antidepressant, and perhaps even an aphrodisiac.

**Increase the challenge.** Find a route that includes hills or stairs. You'll increase muscle strength on the way up and muscle resiliency on the way down, as the tissues absorb minor stretches and strains. If possible, walk in a local park that allows you to go off-road. The bumps, ruts, and changes in surface from dirt to grass to rock will improve your balance and coordination.

**Increase the speed.** The upgrades we've talked about so far improve two key areas of muscular fitness: endurance, which is the ability to repeat movements; and strength, which allows you to generate more force as you climb stairs or ascend a steep hill. Muscle power is another important quality. It allows you to generate force rapidly, and it declines quickly as you get older and do fewer activities that require fast movements.

I'm not talking about sprinting here; that's an advanced form of exercise that I would never recommend to a patient I'm treating for obesity and diabetes. (I don't even think it's come up in conversation.) Nor am I talking about running, which involves high impact on the joints and connective tissues and is extremely risky for someone who's overweight and just getting started. I simply want you to walk faster. There are two ways to do it, both of which are more fun than they sound.

- Time your walks, with the goal of covering your regular distance in less time. Or you can time the first half of your walk and then try to beat that time on the way back. (Just don't cheat by going uphill in the first half and downhill in the second.)

- Mix up your speeds. If you're walking in a city or suburb, you can go faster than your normal pace for one block, then slow down for the next two, and repeat a couple of times. Or you can do more structured intervals, pushing yourself for 30 to 60 seconds and then recovering at a more leisurely pace for 60 to 120 seconds. Over multiple sessions you can cut down the time between intervals until you hit a one-to-one ratio of hard work (you're breathing hard and it *feels* like exercise) and recovery (your breath returns to normal and it feels like an evening stroll).

## BEYOND WALKING

I use outdoor walking as an example because it's so easy and accessible. All you need are clothes and shoes, and the world is your fitness center. But there are lots of ways to get the same results.

**Cardio machines.** You can use every technique I just described on a treadmill, stationary bike, elliptical, or any other machine. You can easily change speeds for intervals and increase resistance or elevation to simulate hills.

**Bicycling.** Riding a bike is slightly more of a challenge than walking, but you can go farther and get there faster. You can even do sprints without much risk to your muscles or joints.

## "Why Did I Wait So Long?"

A lot of my patients are afraid of the gym. Especially the older women. Even if they have a health club membership, they'll use it for swimming, or for walking on a treadmill or riding a stationary bike. Those are all terrific forms of exercise, but nothing can replace the benefits of strength training.

My challenge is to convince those patients to give it a shot.

It usually goes like this.

I ask them to start a walking program or to step up their current routine. They lose a little weight and feel a little better. Then I suggest strength training. I even offer to go into the gym with them the first time to show them how to do the exercises. Not many take me up on it, but a few of them do, and a few others start working with a trainer.

Then something almost magical happens. They do a few dumbbell exercises. Then a few more. They start to get into it. Their strength increases. Their mood improves. They have more energy, more vitality, more "pep," as they like to say. At some point they realize that the simple tasks they used to find so vexing—climbing stairs, lifting groceries, opening a jar—aren't so difficult anymore.

I can't describe how cool it is to see an older woman who came hobbling into my office with a cane walking up to me with longer, faster, steadier strides after a few months in the weight room. Or a patient who'd never even considered lifting weights telling me matter-of-factly how many pushups she can do.

Almost everyone asks herself the same question: "Why didn't I do this earlier? Why did I wait so long?"

**Swimming.** You can gradually build endurance and mix up your speeds. The one higher-effort technique you can't do is swim up hills, unless you're a salmon.

**Fitness classes.** Yoga, spinning, Zumba, Pilates, kickboxing, boot camp—whatever piques your interest is a great choice. Studio cycling classes like spinning have intervals and hill climbs built into the program. With other types of group fitness, you can make progress by . . .

- Improving technique

- Taking more classes

- Taking more advanced classes (or taking classes from instructors known to push a little harder)

- Trying new classes or learning new movement skills outside of class—working with an instructor one-on-one, for example

## PART TWO: STRENGTH TRAINING

Strength exercise works on the principle of *progressive resistance:* When you challenge yourself with increasingly heavy weights, your muscles adapt by getting stronger. It's simple, and at first may even be easy. But the real benefits accrue when it stops being easy, and you begin to understand why the word "resistance" is so important. Overcoming that resistance stimulates a metabolically expensive process in which your muscle tissues remodel themselves by breaking down and then building up.

Higher-effort strength training is purely *anaerobic.* Your muscles can't generate energy the easy way, using a combination of fat and glucose with the help of oxygen from your blood. So they have to do it the hard way, without oxygen, and rely on glucose almost exclusively. This drains glycogen from the working muscles, which your muscles will then have to replace by pulling more glucose from your blood.

But before we get too deep into the process, let's back up a bit and define some terms.

To most people who've never tried it, strength training and bodybuilding are one and the same. It starts early in life: Ask a kid, boy or girl, to "make a muscle," and the kid will immediately flex one or both biceps. Send a 50-year-old man into the gym without a program, and the first thing he'll do is pick up dumbbells and run through every exercise he can think of to work his upper arms. (It might also be the *only* thing he does until he gets some guidance.)

However, the point of strength training isn't to increase the size or enhance the appearance of individual muscles, especially small ones like your biceps. You can worry about that later, if it's important to you. For now, your goal is to improve the functional strength of your entire body. That means focusing on movements.

Not that I'm against building muscles. Outside of my medical practice, it's what I'm known for. It's hard to remember a time when I wasn't a musclehead. So trust me when I say that all your muscles, big and small, will indeed get stronger from the program I'm about to show you. After all, you can't have movements without muscles. You may even notice changes in their appearance. But at this stage those are merely side effects (the good kind).

What you really want is to get stronger systemically. That's why the exercises I recommend mimic basic, natural movement patterns. They may not *feel* natural right away, but the strength you gain most certainly will. Before long you'll find it easier to get up and down, to lift and carry things, and to adjust to life's shifting speeds and random challenges.

## HOME OR HEALTH CLUB?

I work out at home in my garage . . . and my driveway . . . and the street, if necessary. Working out at home is the first choice for many of my patients, as well. Sometimes it's a matter of convenience or finances. Sometimes it's because of social anxiety—a general trepidation about exercising in front of a crowd of presumably judgmental strangers. I get it, and I want to assure you that a good effort will be rewarded, whether you do that work at home or in a commercial fitness center.

However, if you're new to lifting, I *do* recommend joining a low-cost health club for a short time, even if you plan to work out at home. By starting in a gym, you get a chance to try out a variety of equipment and decide what best suits your needs and your budget. You'll also get a sense of how much weight to use for a variety of exercises, something that's really hard to guess when you have no experience. Women will instinctively choose weights that are too light, and men will go the opposite direction—until they realize they can't lift as much as they did back in their prime.

So before I describe the exercises, and how to put them together in a workout, let's look at some of the pros and cons of each choice.

## THE LINGO

**Sets and reps.** These are the basic units of strength training. A rep, short for repetition, means a single execution of an exercise. One pushup is one rep. A set is a series of reps, usually without stopping. So if you're told to do three sets of 10 repetitions (commonly shortened to "three sets of 10," or "3 x 10"), you do the exercise 10 times, rest, do 10 more, rest, and finish by doing 10 more.

**Workout.** This is everything you do in one strength-training session. It typically includes 8 to 10 exercises, each performed for at least one set, along with any exercises you do before and after lifting. A good, comprehensive workout might include a few minutes to warm up, 10 to 20 sets of strength exercises, and something else at the end, like stretching or cardio.

**Program or routine.** Collectively, your workouts are part of a program or routine. So if, a few weeks or months from now, one of your friends asks how you got such impressive results, you can say, "I got my program from Dr. Spencer. You should check it out." Okay, you don't *have* to say it that way, but it would be nice if you did.

## Home-Gym Advantage?

The benefits of home training are obvious enough: your home, your rules. You can work out when you want, wear what you want, and listen to anything you want, all while doing laundry or supervising kids or learning a foreign language. And all without having to worry about who's watching you or what they may be thinking.

## GYM CULTURE FOR THE UNINITIATED

Some of my patients are so intimidated by the thought of entering a gym that I take them there myself to show them it's not such a scary place. It's not like a generation ago, when you were more likely to see a shark in the neighbor's swimming pool than a complete beginner in the local gym—especially one who was middle-aged, overweight, and/or female.

But no matter how newbie-friendly a gym may be, it's still a *gym,* which means it has customs and unwritten codes of etiquette that longtime members expect their fellow lifters to understand and respect. The uninitiated usually don't learn any of these rules until they inadvertently break one. Here are a few faux pas you can easily avoid.

1. **Don't block equipment you aren't using.** It's an innocent mistake: You set your water bottle and towel down on a bench you aren't using. Or you sit on a machine to catch your breath, not realizing someone is waiting for it. Or you stand between two benches to do an exercise that doesn't require either of them, preventing other people from using those benches. The worst violation of all (judging from the number of posts on Facebook complaining about it) is to stand in front of the dumbbell rack to do an exercise. Even if you see others do it, including some who obviously spend a lot of time in the weight room, it's still rude because it

But there's one considerable disadvantage: You'll need equipment. The program doesn't require much to begin with; you can do seven of the nine exercises with just your body weight. But you'll need dumbbells for the other two, and you'll want to use weights on several more as you get stronger.

These days most of my patients have something sitting around, but it often isn't what they need at the moment—it's too heavy or light, or it's mismatched, or it

makes others wait for you to finish before they can use the dumbbells you're blocking.

2. **Be aware of personal space.** In a crowded gym, lifters will arrange themselves in kind of a checkerboard pattern, with everyone facing the mirror. Same with the warmup areas; gym regulars know not to place themselves directly in front of, behind, or alongside someone. You want to give each other a little space to the front, back, and sides. Which leads to the next unwritten rule.

3. **Don't walk in front of people while they're lifting.** It may seem silly to an outsider, but when a lifter stands facing a mirror, all that empty room between her and the mirror is part of her personal space. Walking in front of her, or sliding in between her and someone else, breaks her concentration. So unless you have no choice, you want to walk behind or around people who're in the middle of a set.

4. **Share equipment when asked.** New gym users are sometimes startled by a simple question: "Can I work in?" It might seem like someone's trying to bully or pull rank on you, but it's truly benign. Lifters share equipment all the time. If you're doing multiple sets of an exercise, there's no reason not to let someone work in.

doesn't allow the steady, incremental increases in resistance that you need. To acquire an appropriate range of dumbbells, you have three basic options.

- **Fixed-weight dumbbells.** Preferably, I'd like you to have these in pairs—5, 10, 15, 20 pounds, etc. You may want to start even lighter and go up in smaller increments.

- **Plate-loaded dumbbells.** These usually come with a barbell set. You slide the weights onto the handles and then secure them with collars or clips.

- **Selectorized dumbbells.** These devices allow you to select some or all of their maximum weight, or to select no weight at all and just use the handles. Power Block makes a beginner-friendly pair that goes from 3 to 24 pounds, in 3-pound increments. The most common go up to 50 or more pounds per dumbbell, increasing by 5 pounds at a time. Although they're pricey (well over $100 for a pair), they're compact and easy to use.

Other equipment you can use if you have it, or that you may want to acquire at some point:

- Barbell (it's usually 5 to 7 feet long and requires two hands to lift; I'll show some common barbell exercises in the next chapter)

- Kettlebell (it looks like a bowling ball with a handle)

- Resistance bands (elastic tubing or giant rubber bands)

- Mini-bands (smaller bands that go around your legs)

- Bench (to lie on for chest presses or to elevate your hands or feet for pushup variations)

If you need to purchase equipment before you begin, I recommend casting a wide net. Look at retail prices both on- and offline, as well as resale sites like eBay and Craigslist. The great thing about free weights is that they don't break or wear out, so there's no disadvantage to buying them used. If you buy online, though, beware of shipping costs. Buying new gear with free shipping might be the best deal you'll find.

# Should You Join the Club?

I already noted the biggest advantage of a health club: For a potentially minuscule monthly fee—just $10 a month at Planet Fitness, for example—you get all the equipment you'll ever need. If you live in a city or suburb, you probably have multiple options, which means your biggest challenge is picking the one that you'll use the most and will annoy you the least.

A few suggestions:

- If you don't have any preferences or recommendations, start with one you drive past a lot. Go to the front desk and ask for a walk-through. Because you want a sense of the clientele and atmosphere, try to visit when you're most likely to work out. The early-morning crowd might be very different from the ones who go at noon or in the evening.

- Be sure to check out the locker room, especially if you'll need to shower and change clothes there. There's no guarantee it'll be in the same condition when you actually use it, but if it's skanky on your visit, assume it might be even worse when you're a member.

- Beware of clubs offering shiny objects you're unlikely to use. Pools and saunas are expensive to maintain, and your monthly membership fee will reflect those costs.

- If you like what you see, it's probably worth a trial membership. If you have misgivings, move on to the next gym on your list.

- If all else is equal, to your eyes, you can decide based on whatever criteria matter most to you. Some will choose the cheapest, or the one their friends or neighbors recommend. But you should also consider convenience. You want a gym that's easy to get into and out of. It should be close to home or work, with plenty of parking, and minimal risk of traffic jams eating up your gym time.

# THE WORKOUT

Whether you work out at home or in a gym, your first program includes these exercises.

| | |
|---|---|
| Lower-body strength | Squat, hip raise, split squat |
| Upper-body strength | Pushup or chest press, row, shoulder press, biceps curl (optional) |
| Core stability | Curlup, bird dog, side bridge |

As you can see, there are six or seven strength exercises for your lower and upper body and three stability exercises for your core muscles—the ones in the middle of your body that support your spine. You can do the stability exercises at the beginning or end of your workout, whichever you prefer. I'll explain how (and why) to do them in the next section. First we'll look at the strength exercises.

# Strength Exercises

You'll do one to three sets of 8 to 12 reps of each exercise—one set of each if you're a complete beginner or just pressed for time, and three sets if you're more experienced or ambitious. For most of you, two sets is a good starting point.

Ideally, you'll choose a weight, or an exercise variation, that allows you to work your muscles to fatigue in 9 or 10 reps while maintaining good technique. Fatigue means, "I could do one or two more, but it would be a struggle, and I might have to change my form." When you reach 12 reps on one or more sets, increase the weight or choose a more challenging variation.

# SQUAT

The squat works all the muscles in your lower body, which include the biggest and strongest in your hips and thighs. It's also a movement pattern you use every day when you sit down and stand up.

## BODY-WEIGHT SQUAT

Stand with your feet about shoulder-width apart and your toes pointed straight ahead, or angled out slightly. Raise your arms out in front of you for balance. Push your hips back, like you're going to sit down in a chair, and lower your body as far as you can without discomfort while keeping your heels on the floor. Rise back up to the starting position.

When you can do at least two sets of 12 reps with good form, you'll need to move up to one of the following variations.

### Gym Options?

No machine can replace either the body-weight or goblet squat. But if you have back or knee problems that prevent you from doing them comfortably, you can use the leg press instead.

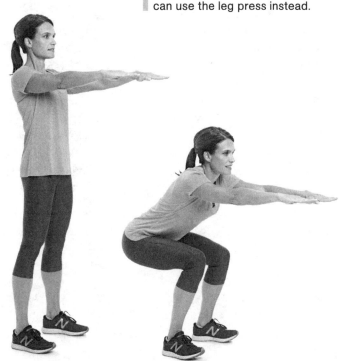

## Other Squat Variations

You can hold dumbbells at arm's length at your sides, or balanced on the edges of your shoulders. The first variation, which was commonly used before the goblet squat (see next page) became popular, has a significant drawback: When you get strong enough to use heavier weights, the gripping muscles in your hands and forearms will give out before your leg muscles. If you have a barbell and want to use it, you can do front or back squats, which I'll explain in the next chapter.

## GOBLET SQUAT

You can use a dumbbell, kettlebell, or weight plate. Whichever you choose, hold the weight with both hands under your chin. Stand with your feet shoulder-width apart, as you did with the body-weight squat. Push your hips back and descend as far as you can, with your heels on the floor and your torso as upright as possible. Return to the starting position.

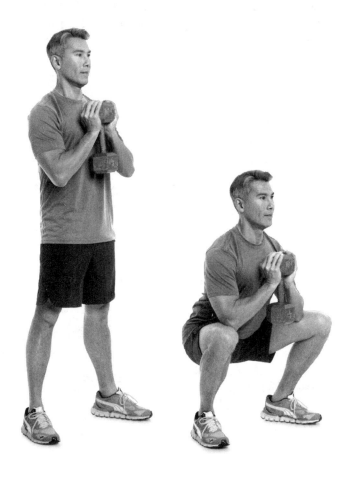

### Progression

Once you have the basic form down and advance to variations like the goblet squat, your strength will increase quickly, and you'll probably surprise yourself with how much weight you can handle. Don't be timid. As long as you don't feel pain in your back or knees, you can really push yourself on this exercise.

# HIP RAISE

This exercise focuses on your seat of power—literally—as you use your gluteal muscles to straighten your hips.

## FLOOR HIP RAISE

Lie on your back with your feet flat on the floor and about 12 inches apart, knees bent, and arms at your sides. Lift your hips until your body forms a straight line from your knees to your chest. Hold for a second or two, feeling the squeeze in your glutes, then lower your hips to the floor and repeat.

### Gym Options?

I understand if you don't want to do the hip raise in a crowded gym. Although there isn't a machine I know of that replicates the movement, feel free to substitute the leg curl if you want. It works the hamstrings (the muscles on the back of your thigh) rather than the glutes, but it's still a good exercise. More advanced lifters can also substitute the deadlift, which I'll explain in the next chapter.

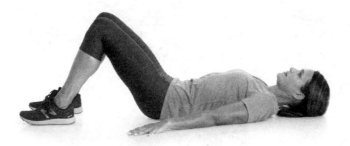

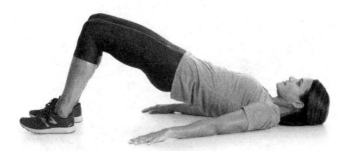

### Progression

You'll quickly max out on the basic version of the hip raise. Here's how to make it more challenging.

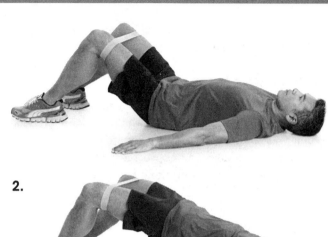

1.  Hold the finishing position of each repetition for 5 to 10 seconds, squeezing your glutes the entire time.

2.  Wear a mini-band around your lower thighs, just above your knees. The band forces you to activate your outer-hip muscles to keep your knees from collapsing inward, which creates a tougher challenge for your glutes.

**2.**

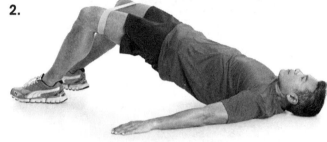

3.  Hold a dumbbell on your lap.

**4.**

4.  Do a single-leg hip raise. Extend one leg, and do all the reps. Rest, and then repeat with the other leg extended. You can count that as one or two sets. Make sure you do the same number of sets and reps with each leg.

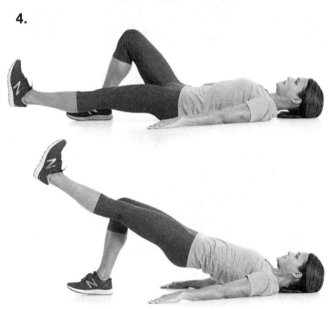

## SPLIT SQUAT

Most of life's movements—walking, running, climbing stairs—require one leg in front of the other. So even though this exercise uses the same muscles as the squat (as you can guess from the name), it uses them in a different way.

### BODY-WEIGHT SPLIT SQUAT

Stand with your feet together and hands behind your head, like you're a prisoner. Take a long step back with one leg, resting your weight on the ball of that foot while keeping your front foot flat on the ground. That's your starting position. Bend your knees as you lower your body, keeping your torso upright. Ideally, your rear knee will come within an inch or two of the floor, but don't try to push yourself beyond your pain-free range of motion. Return to the starting position and do all the reps. Switch legs and repeat. You can count that as one or two sets. Just make sure you do the same number of sets and reps with each leg.

### Gym Options?

At home or in the gym, you should do split squats or lunges as described, first with body weight and then with some kind of external load. As with the hip thrust, there isn't a machine that uses the same muscles in the same movement pattern.

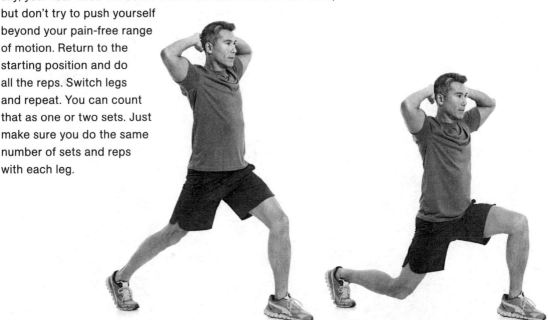

### Lunge

If you find the split squat easy, you can try the lunge. Stand with your feet together, and either step back with one leg into a reverse lunge (the easier variation), or forward into a traditional lunge (which can be a little tougher on the knees). In either version, lower your body until your rear knee nearly touches the floor, then straighten your body as you step back to the starting position, with your feet together. You can use any of the loading options I describe on the next page.

## WEIGHTED SPLIT SQUAT

When you can do multiple sets of 12 reps
with each leg, it's time to add some weight.
Your options:

1. Hold a single dumbbell, kettlebell, or
   weight plate in the goblet position.

2. Hold two dumbbells at arm's length at your
   sides.

3. Hold a single dumbbell at your shoulder.
   Hold it with your left hand at your left
   shoulder if you're stepping back with your
   right leg, and vice versa.

**1.**

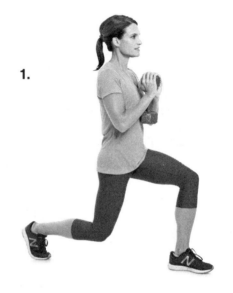

**2.**

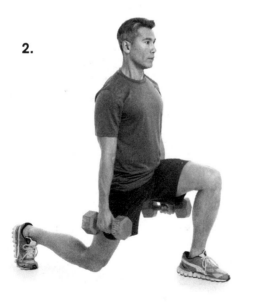

**3.**

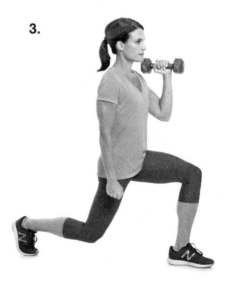

# PUSHUP OR CHEST PRESS

This is the first of two pressing exercises; it works your chest, shoulders, and triceps muscles. I hope you'll use the pushup if possible, at least to start the program. It activates a lot of muscles in your upper back and core to stabilize your body throughout the movement. But it's also an extremely challenging exercise for heavier people. So if you can't do it comfortably or with good form, or if you simply prefer the chest press, by all means go with what works best for you.

## PUSHUP

In the traditional pushup, you position yourself with your hands and toes on the floor, your arms straight, your hands about shoulder-width apart, and your body in a straight line from your neck through your ankles. Bend your elbows and lower your body, stopping when your chest is a couple of inches from the floor or you can't go any farther. Push back up to the starting position, keeping your body straight all the way down and all the way back up.

## Gym Options?

Any commercial health club should have one or more chest press machines. Most will also have a device called the Smith machine, a barbell on rails that moves along a fixed vertical path. Fitness professionals don't like the Smith machine for presses because it doesn't allow the bar to move in its natural trajectory, which isn't straight up and down. However, the Smith is a great option for elevated push-ups. It's sturdy enough to support a body of any size, and it allows you to lower the bar as you get stronger.

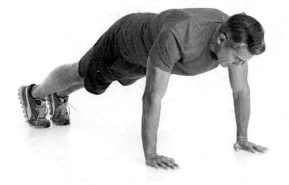
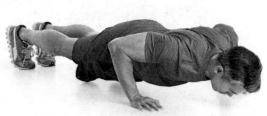

### ELEVATED PUSHUP

If the traditional pushup isn't an option—
either because you don't yet have the
strength for it, or your body simply won't
allow it—the next option is to elevate your
hands. You can set them on a low box, rest
them against a wall, or choose any angle in
between. The form is exactly the same:
Lower and raise your body as a unit, keeping it straight from neck to ankles.

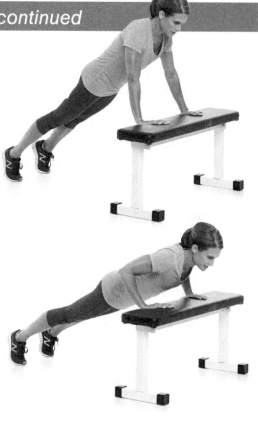

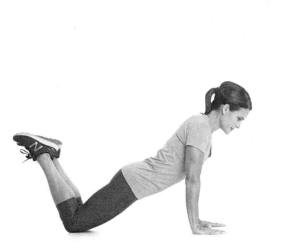

### BENT-KNEE PUSHUP

Get into a modified pushup position, with
your weight resting on your knees instead
of your toes. Everything else is the same.

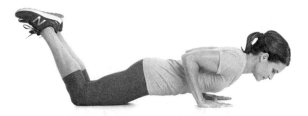

### Pushup Progression

When you can do multiple sets of 12 pushups, you should make it more challenging, no matter which
variation you started with. On elevated pushups, you make progress by doing your sets with your
hands closer to the floor. If you're doing traditional pushups and they're already on the floor, make it
harder by elevating your feet on a box, step, or bench.

## DUMBBELL CHEST PRESS

Lie on your back on a bench holding a pair of dumbbells straight up over your chest. Spread your legs and set your feet on the floor. Make sure the back of your head, upper back, and glutes rest on the bench, with a slight arch in your lower back. Bend your elbows and lower the weights until your upper arms are level with your torso. Push the weights back up to the starting position.

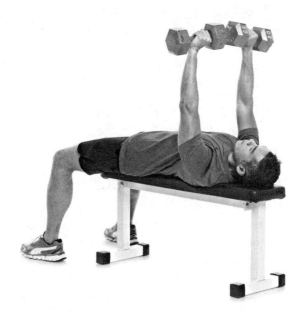

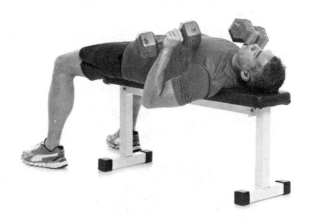

### Chest Press Variations

If you have a bench that allows it, you can do an incline chest press, with the top part of the bench elevated 30 to 45 degrees. You can also do a barbell chest press on a flat or inclined bench.

# ROW

I would run out of fingers, and possibly other appendages, counting the many ways to do rowing exercises. I'll include the most common and accessible below, and a couple more in the next chapter. All of them do the same basic thing: work the muscles of the upper back, along with the biceps. Most also activate shoulder and core muscles.

## SINGLE-ARM DUMBBELL ROW, FREESTANDING

With a dumbbell in your right hand, stand with your left foot forward, knee bent, and your left hand resting on your thigh, just above the knee. Bend forward so your torso is at a 45-degree angle to the floor and your right arm hangs straight down from your shoulder. Pull the weight to the side of your torso, then slowly lower it to the starting position. Keep your shoulders square to the floor throughout the exercise—don't allow your upper body to rotate, in other words. Do all your reps, then switch sides and repeat. That's one set.

## Gym Options?

Cable machines may be the best argument for working out in a health club. You can do seated or standing rows, using a variety of attachments that work your back in slightly different ways. You can also do lat pulldowns, in which you pull a bar down to your chest. Aside from the cable stations, most gyms will also have machines that mimic the row, pulldown, and pullup or chinup. All of those devices give you the option of rowing with an underhand grip, which gives your biceps more work.

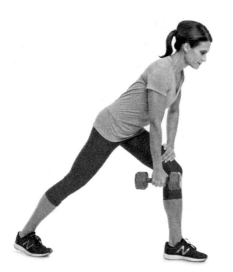 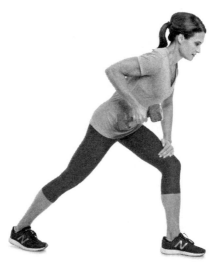

## SINGLE-ARM DUMBBELL ROW, HAND SUPPORTED

Set a dumbbell on the floor next to a sturdy bench or step that's about 18 to 24 inches high. Bend forward at your hips, keeping your back straight, and rest one hand on the bench. Pick up the dumbbell with the other hand, and start with your arm hanging straight down from your shoulder. Pull the dumbbell up to the side of your torso, again without rotating your shoulders. Do all your reps, then switch sides and repeat. That's one set.

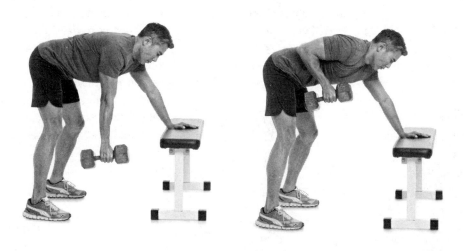

### Other Variations

You can do rows with a resistance band attached to something sturdy, using one or both arms. You can also use a barbell, although it can be pretty tough on your lower back.

## SHOULDER PRESS

This is the second pressing exercise, and it works some of the same muscles in your shoulders and triceps. It's just a different angle—overhead instead of straight off your chest. But it's still an important movement pattern, especially if you're deskbound and don't have many opportunities to lift something overhead. You need a full and friction-free range of motion not just in your arms, but in the entire complex of bones and joints in your upper torso, including (and perhaps especially) the shoulder blades. That's exactly what the shoulder press does.

### DUMBBELL SHOULDER PRESS

Stand holding a dumbbell in each hand just above your shoulders, with your palms turned toward each other. Set your feet about shoulder-width apart. Press the weights straight overhead, pause, and lower them to the starting position.

### Gym Options?

Gyms typically have a shoulder press machine. It's an okay choice if you prefer it to free weights. But I want to throw out a few words of caution. Most machines I've seen force you to lift with both arms locked in a fixed trajectory. Human shoulders don't work that way; they're structured to allow independent actions. We tend to be dominant on one side, and develop muscular and postural differences to allow us to express more strength and force with that side. That's why I prefer dumbbells. Your arms can choose the best path, which might be slightly different on each side. Forcing them onto the same path can lead to injuries over time.

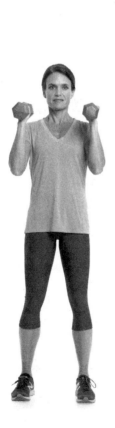
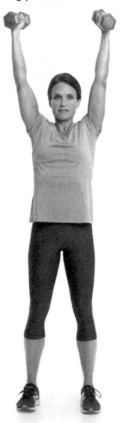

## Variations

- You can do the shoulder press while standing or sitting. I recommend standing, but if you feel unsteady or find yourself leaning back to keep your balance, you'll probably do better if you sit on a sturdy bench or step.

- You can hold the weights with your palms facing out, if that feels more natural than having your palms in. Or you can pick an angle somewhere in between. Choose whichever allows a comfortable, friction-free range of motion.

- Finally, you can do a single-arm shoulder press. The key is to maintain the same form and posture you'd use with two dumbbells. No bending, leaning, or twisting, in other words. Doing all the reps with each arm constitutes a single set.

- The barbell shoulder press is a more technically complex lift. If you need or prefer to use it in this program, you can find instructions in Chapter 13.

## A Note about Weight Selection

It's okay to start with light weights for your first few workouts. They should certainly be lighter than the weight you use for the row, since that exercise involves much bigger and stronger muscles in your upper back. Your goal at first, as I said, is a smooth and painless range of motion. But once you master the movement pattern, don't be afraid to go a little heavier.

# BICEPS CURL (OPTIONAL)

As I mentioned earlier, the biceps curl is the one strength exercise that everyone knows how to do, and everyone assumes they're *supposed* to do. But it's not an especially important movement. How many people do you know—young or old, weak or strong—who can't bend their elbows? Compare that to the number who would struggle to do a squat with good form. You can use it or skip it in this program. Your choice.

## DUMBBELL BICEPS CURL

Stand holding two dumbbells with your arms at your sides, palms facing forward. Pull your shoulders down, like you're standing at attention. Bend your elbows and curl the weights straight up toward your shoulders. Pause long enough to feel the squeeze in your biceps, then lower the weights. Keep your shoulders down throughout the movement, and don't allow your torso to lean forward or back.

### Gym Options?

Gyms have curl machines, for reasons that escape me. I've used them from time to time, but I don't think I've seen one that was an improvement on free-weight variations. (And trust me, I've done a *lot* of curls in my day.) However, gyms usually have an EZ-curl bar: a shorter, lighter barbell that you can hold with your hands angled inward, which is much easier on your wrists. You can also do curls with cable machines, using a variety of different attachments and grips.

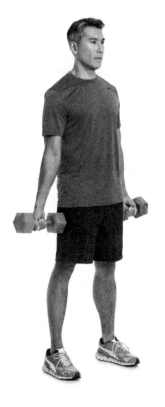
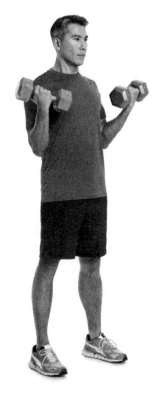

## Variations

- Start with your palms facing in, and then twist them outward as you lift, a movement called *supination*.

- Keep them facing in throughout the movement, a variation called the hammer curl. Your arms are stronger in this position, so you can use heavier weights.

- Curl with one arm at a time, alternating so one descends as the other rises. But don't bend or twist your torso as you alternate. (In other words, don't try to emulate the pictures you see in bodybuilding magazines, with the models straining to admire their biceps veins.)

- The barbell curl is also an option, but not one I recommend. It puts a lot of strain on your wrists and elbows.

# Stability Exercises

These three exercises come from Stuart McGill, PhD, professor of spine biomechanics at the University of Waterloo in Canada. Dr. McGill—Stu to his many friends in the fitness and medical professions—has spent his career studying back pain. His studies have shown that the "big three" exercises, as he calls them, can both alleviate back pain for those who have it and prevent pain in those who don't. They do that by developing the midbody muscles that provide spinal stability—keeping your lower back in a safe, natural position.

So why not just have you do situps and crunches for your abdominal muscles? Dr. McGill's research shows that the repetitive spine bending of the situp will create an injury, sooner or later. And the bigger muscles you develop with the crunch don't actually promote spinal stability. Stability comes from a combination of strength, muscular endurance, and movement coordination. Stronger muscles provide more protection than weaker ones. Endurance protects your spine because you can maintain your posture longer while standing, sitting, or moving around. Coordination prevents you from hurting yourself when making the sudden, unanticipated movements that life sometimes requires.

One caution: If you work out early in the morning, you want to do these exercises at the end, when your body is thoroughly warmed up. Your spinal disks accumulate fluid overnight (this is why you're slightly taller in the morning), which drains back to normal levels after a little time out of bed and on your feet. The fluid creates greater-than-normal pressure on the disks, which makes it risky to do core exercises right after you get out of bed.

# CURLUP

Lie on your back on the floor, with your left leg straight, right knee bent, and right foot flat on the floor. Place both hands, palms down, on the floor beneath your lower back, and then lift your elbows slightly. The back of your head, upper back, palms, and glutes all rest on the floor, along with the back of your left leg and your right foot. From that starting position, raise your head and shoulders *slightly*. Hold for 10 seconds, and return to the starting position. That's one repetition. Do four to six reps per set. You can switch legs on each set if you want, but it's not necessary.

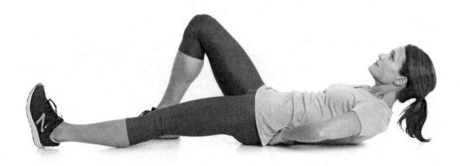

## Tips

Dr. McGill suggests that you imagine your head is resting on a scale that's level with the floor; you want to raise your head and shoulders just enough for the scale to go to zero. Keep your head and neck in the exact same alignment. Tucking your chin to raise your head creates unnecessary strain on your neck.

## BIRD DOG

Get down on all fours, with your hands directly beneath your shoulders and your knees below your hips. Slowly extend your left arm and right leg until they're parallel to the floor and in line with your torso and neck. Hold for 10 seconds, then pull them back to the starting position. Now extend your right arm and left leg, hold 10 seconds, and pull them back. Try for three reps with each arm and leg extended. If you hold each rep for 10 seconds, a set will take just over a minute.

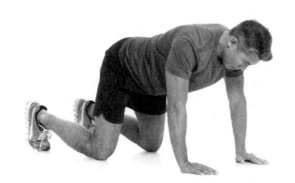

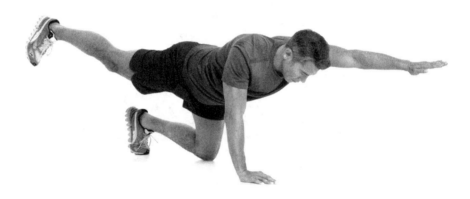

### Tips

- *Actively* push your arm and leg away from your torso when you extend your limbs, and deliberately pull them back, rather than letting them drop to the floor.

- When your limbs are fully extended, they should be aligned with your torso and on the same plane. You don't want an arm or a leg rising above or lingering below.

- Your hips should stay parallel to the floor throughout the movement. That'll be a challenge at first, especially if you've never done this exercise. One side will probably rise higher than the other. To keep your hips down, try flexing your foot as you extend your leg, as if you're pointing your heel at someone standing behind you.

## SIDE BRIDGE *(BEGINNER)*

Lie on your left side with your knees and hips bent. Your weight rests on your left elbow and the outside of your left leg from the knee to the edge of your foot. Your right leg is on top of your left. You can rest your right hand on your right hip or your left shoulder, whichever is more comfortable. That's your starting position. Push your hips forward so your body is in a straight line from your nose through your torso, pelvis, and knees, with your upper back on a plane that's perpendicular to the floor, as if you had a wall right behind you. Hold for 10 seconds while breathing normally, then push your hips back to the starting position. That's one rep. Do three or four reps, then switch sides and repeat. That's one set, which should be plenty your first few workouts.

When you can do one or more sets of up to six reps per side (keeping in mind that six reps means you're holding the position for a total of 1 minute per side), it's time to try the more challenging version.

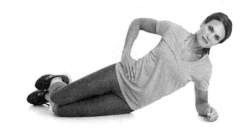

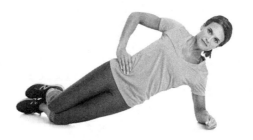

## SIDE BRIDGE

This time, lie on your side with your weight resting on your left elbow and forearm and the outside of your left foot. Your right foot can rest on your left, as shown, or slightly ahead of it on the floor. Lift your hips off the floor so your body forms a straight line from your nose through the center of your torso and pelvis, with your back perpendicular to the floor. You can rest your right hand on your left shoulder or your right hip. (The latter is slightly more challenging.) Hold for 10 seconds, breathing normally, then lower your body. That's one rep. Do four to six reps, switch sides, and repeat.

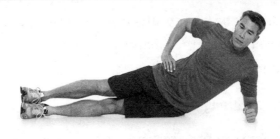

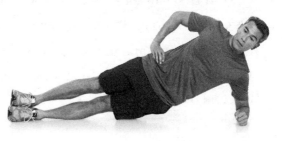

# HOW TO WORK OUT

I've thrown a lot of instructions and numbers at you, so let's clarify exactly what I mean. Here's what the program looks like in a simple chart.

| EXERCISE | SETS | REPS |
|---|---|---|
| Squat | 1–3 | 8–12 |
| Hip raise | 1–3 | 8–12 |
| Split squat | 1–3 | 8–12* |
| Pushup or chest press | 1–3 | 8–12 |
| Row | 1–3 | 8–12* |
| Shoulder press | 1–3 | 8–12 |
| Biceps curl (optional) | 1–3 | 8–12 |
| Curlup | 1–2 | See page 169 |
| Bird dog | 1–2 | See page 170 |
| Side bridge | 1–2 | See page 171 |

*Each side

## Frequency

You'll get the best results if you use this program two or three times a week, with at least 48 hours in between each workout. The classic schedule is Monday-Wednesday-Friday.

## Reps for Strength Exercises

- For your first workout, take your best guess at appropriate starting weights or exercise variations. Shoot for about 10 reps of each exercise.

- If you get started and immediately realize the weight is too heavy or the variation is too challenging, stop the set. Select a lighter weight or easier variation, and try again.

- Conversely, if it's too easy, and you aren't challenged enough, stop at 12 reps and regard it as a warmup set. Select a heavier weight or more advanced variation, and do another set.

- If you can do eight or nine reps, use that same weight or variation for subsequent workouts, with the goal of increasing reps.

- Once you get to 12 reps, you can either increase the weight or challenge, or add an extra set with that same weight or variation.

## Sets for Strength Exercises

- The first time you work out, you may need to do multiple sets of each exercise just to figure out the best starting point.

- You'll know you have the right weight or variation when you reach 10 reps and feel that you could *maybe* do one or two more, but not necessarily with good form.

- Always stop a set when you feel your form change and you have to "cheat" by bending your back or shortening the range of motion.

- Most readers will do best with two sets of each exercise, versus one. Your body will make faster adaptations to the program, and you'll get more total exercise.

- If you choose to do three sets, you can use the first one as a warmup, doing 8 to 10 reps with a lighter weight. Follow it with two challenging sets.

## Rest for Strength Exercises

- You'll need a short break between exercises, or between multiple sets of the same exercise. Thirty seconds is a typical rest period.

- If you don't feel you need a break, you probably aren't pushing yourself hard enough. Anaerobic exercise creates a shortage of oxygen, and it usually takes a few deep breaths at the end of a set to let your body catch up. A good set should also fatigue the working muscles. So if you can do two sets of the same exercise without rest, you're probably using, at most, half the weight you should be lifting, or doing a much easier variation than you can handle.

- Try not to sit down between sets, unless you're so short of breath you need to. (And if you are that short of breath, you're probably pushing *too* hard.) Use that time to set up for the next set or exercise.

## Reps, Sets, and Rest Periods for Stability Exercises

- For each repetition of the curlup, bird dog, and side bridge, you'll hold the position for up to 10 seconds.

- It doesn't have to be *exactly* 10 seconds, of course. Counting to 10 is fine. Your focus should be on the position, rather than the clock.

- Breathe normally while holding. The last thing you want to do is repeatedly hold your breath for 10 seconds at a time.

- A good set might be just three or four reps. Six reps—60 seconds of holding the position—is the maximum.

- One set of each exercise should be plenty to start with. (Keep in mind that the side bridge requires an equal number of reps for each side.)

- Take as much rest as you need between sets, or when switching sides on the side bridge.

# Alternating Exercises

To use your time more efficiently, you can try combinations of exercises for different muscle groups. You would do a set of one exercise, a set of the other, rest, and repeat one or two times. Or you could do a set of one, rest, do a set of the other, rest, and continue like that. Your pairings could work as shown in the following chart.

| EXERCISE | SETS | REPS |
|---|---|---|
| 1a. Squat | 1–3 | 8–12 |
| 1b. Pushup or chest press | 1–3 | 8–12 |
| 2a. Hip raise | 1–3 | 8–12 |
| 2b. Row | 1–3 | 8–12* |
| 3a. Split squat | 1–3 | 8–12* |
| 3b. Shoulder press | 1–3 | 8–12 |
| 3c. Biceps curl (optional) | 1–3 | 8–12 |
| 4a. Curlup | 1–2 | See page 169 |
| 4b. Bird dog | 1–2 | See page 170 |
| 4c. Side bridge | 1–2 | See page 171 |

*Each side

# WARMUP

It's a good idea to give your body a chance to warm up a little before lifting. There are three components to a warmup.

1. A general warmup—a few minutes of walking, riding a stationary bike, or doing some jumping jacks or a little shadow boxing—will raise your heart rate and your core temperature. This increases bloodflow and makes any type of activity a little smoother and easier.

2. Mobility exercises—moving your arms and legs through a range of motion as you would with lunges and arm circles—will help prepare your joints for the movements in the workout.

3. Warmup sets, using a lighter weight or easier variation, will prepare your muscles and joints for the specific challenges of the exercise you're about to perform.

Do you need to do all three steps? No. At first, you just need to not be cold. So if you exercise early in the morning, or in a chilly basement or garage, or after spending time outside in the dead of winter, you want to spend a few minutes doing something to get the blood flowing and help your muscles loosen up. As you get more ambitious, and you start pushing heavier weights, then you want to spend a little more time preparing your body for the challenge.

## FINISHING OFF

After you finish these exercises, if you feel like doing a little more, you can throw in a few stretches, or add some cardio exercise, indoors or out.

## PUTTING IT ALL TOGETHER

Careful readers will notice that I've done exactly what I criticized in Chapter 4: I've given you a to-do list that includes 30 minutes of walking every day and two to three strength workouts a week. It would be great if you did that much exercise. But I don't expect you to. Instead, I hope you'll mix and match to get a range of benefits without overwhelming yourself with the details.

**Every day of the week.** Please do something. A short walk after dinner. A stroll around the park while your kids or grandkids practice soccer. Any sort of movement is better than none.

**Most days of the week.** Some kind of deliberate physical activity for at least a half hour, preferably after dinner or another meal.

**Two or three days a week.** Something that pushes you a bit. It could be strength training, or a group-exercise class at your gym or community center, or just a daily walk that's longer or faster than usual.

So a weekly schedule might look something like this.

*Monday:* strength workout, exercise class, or longer walk after dinner

*Tuesday:* half-hour walk after lunch or dinner

*Wednesday:* strength workout, exercise class, or fast walk after dinner

*Thursday:* half-hour walk after lunch or dinner

**Friday:** strength workout, exercise class, or challenging walk (hills, stairs, trail) after dinner

**Saturday:** chores or shopping

**Sunday:** leisurely walk or bike ride with family or friends

Notice how many times I used "or"? You don't need to check off every item on the list to get the lifesaving, diabetes-reversing benefits of exercise. Just aim for something every day, and something a little more challenging a few times a week.

# THE PLANET FITNESS WORKOUT

If you belong to a health club like Planet Fitness, or have access to a reasonably well-equipped company gym or community center, you can make a strength workout incredibly simple with this combination of (mostly) machine exercises.

1. **Leg press**

2. **Chest press**

3. **Seated row**

4. **Leg curl**

5. **Shoulder press***

6. **Lat pulldown**

*As noted earlier, I recommend using dumbbells instead of a machine for the shoulder press.

Do two or three sets of 8 to 12 reps, using the parameters I described earlier: Shoot for about 10 good reps per set, and when you can do 12, increase the weight. You can do "straight sets," finishing all the sets of one exercise before moving on to the next, or a circuit, doing one set of each exercise and then repeating the sequence once or twice.

## CHAPTER 13

# Going Longer, Getting Stronger

**WAY BACK IN CHAPTER 1,** I warned you that I'm going to talk a lot about exercise, but not in the way you might expect: "The goal isn't to turn you into a marathoner or mountain climber or bodybuilder. . . . [W]e'll start where you are, with the goal of doing just a little more. If you're not doing anything, a little more than zero is pretty easy."

That's exactly what we covered in Chapter 4—how to do more than zero. By the end of Chapter 12, we were talking about a *lot* more than zero. I proposed a simple and reasonable plan for staying active 7 days a week: Three days a week, you'll do a strength workout, take an exercise class, or go for a longer, faster, or more challenging walk. You'll do a shorter walk 2 days a week, and on weekends you'll do something obligatory (errands and chores) and something pleasant and social. The particulars of what you do and when you do it don't matter as much as the fact that you're up and moving for at least a while every day of the week, and a few times you're doing something that pushes you just a bit outside your comfort zone.

But careful readers will notice that there's an ellipsis in the opening paragraph, and they may wonder what I left out. Here it is.

"If you *want* to do any of those things, great; this book could very well get you started down that path."

I haven't changed my mind. This chapter isn't for those who aspire to extreme accomplishments, like completing a marathon or triathlon. My goal is to address those of you who are already doing exercise programs that are somewhat more ambitious than what we've talked about so far, along with those of you who do so well on the program in Chapter 12 that you want to know what's next.

So now it's time to talk about the benefits of going beyond basic physical activity and working to increase what your body is capable of doing. I'll approach it two different ways: increasing your cardiovascular fitness, and increasing your strength and muscle quality. Both are linked to what we call healthspan—not just a longer life, but more years of active, healthy *living,* with fewer disabilities and limitations.

An aggressive approach to either outcome—higher cardiovascular fitness or strength—can get you to more or less the same place. Which you choose should be dictated by what you enjoy and what your body naturally adapts to. Those may or may not be the same thing.

For example, some of my male patients are naturally big guys. Like me, they may have had some success in sports like football or wrestling in high school or college. Once they get back in the weight room, they see fast and steady gains, which increases their motivation to work out. If I pushed those guys to focus on cardio, improvements would be slower, frustration would mount, and they'd be more likely to give up.

Conversely, not many of my female patients were encouraged to participate in sports in their early years, especially those who have been heavy most of their lives. Exercise may have been used as punishment, or something others tried to shame them into doing. If they can get past that baggage, and discover that they *like* to move, and that it's kind of cool to be stronger, they see a whole world of unexplored potential. But because they don't have the time or energy for "all of the above," they tend to gravitate toward whatever best fits their comfort level. Some pursue strength training because it's something they can do at home. Others want to do what their friends are doing.

There's no right or wrong choice. My goal here is to help you get the most out of whatever you choose.

## HIGHER (AEROBIC) POWER

Exercise scientists have a few ways to measure what a body is capable of doing. You may have heard of $VO_2$ max, for example. It's a common way to describe aerobic capacity—how hard you can push yourself while still using oxygen to help your muscles generate energy. To many of my fellow doctors and health experts, aerobic fitness is fitness, period.

But real life includes a mix of aerobic and anaerobic challenges. You can rank those challenges with a measure called metabolic equivalent of task, or MET. Sitting still is a 1 MET activity. Walking at a fairly brisk 4-mile-per-hour pace is 5 METs. Jogging at a 10-minute-mile pace is 10 METs. The highest recorded performance ever, 26 METs, was by a 22-year-old cross-country skier.

Here's why METs matter.

Five METs is considered the red line. If you can't manage a 5-MET task, like walking a mile in 15 minutes, you're at much higher risk for an early grave. Increase your capacity by 1 MET and you lower your risk of premature death by 12 percent. A 2-MET improvement lowers your risk by 24 percent, and so on, up to 10 METs, which is the highest fitness level linked to longevity. (If you can get beyond 10 METs, it's unlikely that you'd be one of my patients.)

Before I give you a list of activities and their MET values, I want to reiterate my biggest point: All movement is good. Walking at a normal pace has benefits. Same with taking a yoga class or doing a light workout in your basement. Even if something you enjoy doesn't increase your fitness level, it at least prevents it from getting worse. As long as you give yourself the option to reach that higher capacity, it'll be there when you're ready to try for it. Now turn the page to see that list of MET values.

# MET VALUES OF COMMON ACTIVITIES

| ACTIVITY | METS |
|---|---|
| Around the House and Yard | |
| Sitting at a desk and working on a computer | 1.5 |
| Sexual intercourse (enthusiastic) | 1.5 |
| Light housework (cooking, etc.) | 2–2.5 |
| Playing a musical instrument | 2–2.5 |
| Cleaning, mopping, sweeping, vacuuming | 3–4 |
| Gardening, weeding, mowing lawn | 4–5 |
| Home repair and construction | 5–6 |
| Digging, shoveling snow, chopping wood, moving furniture | 6 |
| Outdoor Exercise | |
| Walking 3 mph (20-minute miles) | 3.3 |
| Riding a bike, leisurely pace (below 10 mph) | 4 |
| Walking 4 mph (15-minute miles) | 5 |
| Riding a bike, moderate pace (10–12 mph) | 6 |
| Walking 4.5 mph (13-minute miles) | 6.3 |
| Hiking and backpacking | 6–7 |
| Walking uphill | 6–7 |
| Walking uphill with a 30-pound load | 8 |
| Riding a bike, serious effort (12–14 mph) | 8 |
| Running 5 mph (12-minute miles) | 8 |
| Riding a bike, really pushing it (14–16 mph) | 10 |
| Running 6 mph (10-minute miles) | 10 |
| Running 6.7 mph (9-minute miles) | 11 |
| Running up stairs | 15 |
| Indoor Exercise | |
| Strength training, very light (dumbbells or machines) | 3* |
| Yoga | 3* |

| Indoor Exercise (cont.) | |
| --- | --- |
| Water aerobics | 4 |
| Stationary cycling, easy (100 watts†) | 5.5 |
| Strength training, pushing yourself (mostly free weights) | 6* |
| Stationary cycling, moderate effort (150 watts†) | 7 |
| Stationary rowing, moderate effort (100 watts†) | 7 |
| Swimming laps, moderate effort (50 yards a minute) | 8 |
| Stationary rowing, pushing yourself (150 watts†) | 8.5 |
| Stationary cycling, maximum effort (200 watts†) | 10.5 |
| Sports and Recreation‡ | |
| Bowling or horseshoes | 3 |
| Golf | 3.5–4.5 |
| Hunting or fishing | 3–6 |
| Dancing | 4.5 |
| Shooting baskets | 4.5 |
| Tennis (doubles) | 5 |
| Baseball or softball | 5 |
| Kayaking | 5 |
| Downhill skiing | 5–7 |
| Boxing (hitting a bag) | 6 |
| Tennis (singles) | 8 |
| Competitive team sports (basketball, hockey, volleyball, etc.) | 8 |
| Soccer | 10 |

*Anyone who's taken a yoga class will tell you that each style has its own pace, and each teacher has her own ideas about how hard to push students. Similarly, if you've observed a variety of people working out with weights, you know there's no single intensity level that everyone uses. So don't take these MET values as the final word. If it feels like you're working harder than the indicated level, you probably are.

†Watts are a measure of power output that most stationary bikes will keep track of, along with speed, distance, resistance level, and time. How hard it is to crank the pedals—and thus how many watts of power you generate—will vary at different speeds and resistance levels.

‡Obviously, there are many ways to do these activities, and your individual effort on any given day will vary by your experience, skill level, competition, and the conditions of the field or venue.

## How (and Why) to Reach the Next Level

The simplest way to gain a MET is to do an activity you enjoy and get progressively better at it. This might be a logical progression for you.

- You start walking every day.

- One day a week, you walk 3 miles in an hour (3.3 METs).

- You gradually increase your speed, until you can walk 4 miles in an hour (5 METs).

- You find a route that includes a long, steep hill (6 METs).

- After a year of walking almost every day, you tackle that hill while wearing a 30-pound backpack (8 METs).

That may seem impossibly ambitious to you right now. But let's say that over the course of the year, you also lose some weight. It's amazing how fast your performance improves while your weight falls. You can go longer, farther, and faster, and feel better afterward. There's nothing more motivating than the sense of accomplishment you get when your hard work results in measurable improvements in something that matters to you.

But if you're looking for the fastest and most direct way to improve your fitness, you can't do better than high-intensity interval training (HIIT). The concept, which I explained in Chapter 12, is simple: You go hard for a defined period (usually 30 to 60 seconds), slow down for another period (usually 60 to 120 seconds), and repeat several times. With a relatively short workout—perhaps 15 to 20 minutes, three times a week—you can achieve benefits equal to, if not surpassing, those from much longer cardio workouts done at a steady pace.

Here's a sample interval program, which you can try with any type of endurance exercise, from walking to swimming to shadow boxing.

- Warm up for about 5 minutes, gradually increasing the intensity (on a stationary bike, for example, you might go from level 1 up to level 4).

- Go hard for 30 seconds (perhaps level 8 on a stationary bike).

- Recover for 60 seconds (level 2 or 3 on the bike).

- Do a total of four intervals your first workout.

- After the final interval, which includes 60 seconds of recovery, you can cool down for another minute or two at an even easier pace, if you want.

With the optional 2-minute cooldown at the end, it'll take a total of 13 minutes. You can add one interval a week until you're doing a total of eight per workout. Increase the cooldown at the end to 3 minutes, and it'll take 20 minutes altogether.

If you reach that point, you can mix it up by lengthening the intervals to 45 or 60 seconds; shortening the recovery period until you're doing a one-to-one ratio of work to recovery; or some combination.

Cap each session at 20 minutes, with a maximum of three a week and a day of recovery in between. Unless you're a competitive athlete, those are probably the upper limits for HIIT workouts.

## THE STRONG LIVE LONG

As I mentioned earlier, when my fellow doctors talk about fitness as it applies to health (as opposed to aesthetics or athletic performance), the conversation almost always begins and ends with aerobic fitness. It shouldn't. We've known for a while that strength and mortality are intimately linked. Stronger people tend to live longer, with less risk of disability, compared to those who are weaker.

The studies linking strength to longevity are usually done with a simple handgrip test, and admittedly it isn't the best measure of total-body strength. By comparison, a VO$_2$ max test on a treadmill will give you a much better snapshot of someone's aerobic fitness. But even with that limitation, there's a very good track record of handgrip strength predicting longevity. In one massive study that followed 140,000 men and women in 17 countries for at least 4 years, better grip strength was correlated with a lower risk of heart disease, stroke, and death from any cause. (There was also a trend toward a lower diabetes risk among the strongest, although it wasn't statistically significant.)

A study at the Cooper Clinic in Dallas looked beyond grip strength, but only in men. The researchers found that those with the most upper- and lower-body strength, adjusted for age and body weight, had the lowest risk of death from heart disease, cancer, or any other cause. (They used bench press and leg press machines to measure strength.)

We can only speculate about why stronger people achieve some degree of protec-

## ANOTHER REASON TO TAKE YOUR FITNESS UP A NOTCH

Every winter, hundreds of people have fatal heart attacks while shoveling snow from their driveways. Why snow? If you'll pardon the cliché (and the pun), it's the perfect storm for catching people at their most vulnerable.

In a normal workout, you give yourself a chance to warm up before you do anything strenuous. The warmup elevates your core temperature and gets a little adrenaline flowing, which opens up your blood vessels. Snow shoveling reverses all those dynamics. You typically shovel your driveway in the morning, when your body temperature is relatively low, and the cold weather restricts your blood vessels. On top of all that, you don't start out with lighter activities; you jump right into the heaviest part of the task, lifting and throwing 10 to 20 pounds of snow at a time, and you keep going until you've finished the job . . . or the job has finished you.

Snow isn't the only challenge life might throw your way. You may need to push a stalled car, or carry an injured child, or do *something* that puts a sudden load on your cardiovascular system.

You'll never know if your fitness routine saved your life in those circumstances. But it sure is nice to know you can get through them without fear.

tion against the major causes of death. There's certainly a chicken-and-egg aspect to the question. Are healthier people more likely to be strong? Sure. And are stronger people more likely to be healthy? Absolutely. So which comes first, strength or health? Do you have to be healthy before you start working out, or does working out make you healthy? I don't know, and it may be a different answer for each of us. All I can say with confidence is that it's good to be strong.

## How to Get Stronger

The program in Chapter 12 showed you how to get started. This intermediate-level program uses many of the same exercises, but it's more aggressive. You'll work out four times a week, instead of three. And instead of doing total-body workouts each time, you'll alternate between workouts for upper- and lower-body muscles. In gym lingo, these are called split routines. The rationale?

If you do the maximum three sets of each strength exercise I listed in Chapter 12, including the optional biceps curls, that's 21 total sets. Add in a warmup at the beginning and the stability exercises at the end, and you're looking at a pretty challenging workout. But for many of you, it might be both too much and too little training.

Let's start with the "too little" part: If all else is equal, the more work you do for each muscle group, the more your strength and muscle quality will improve. You can do more total work if you spread it across four workouts, instead of packing it all into three. Plus, by splitting upper- and lower-body exercises into separate workouts, and working each muscle group twice a week instead of three times, you give all your muscles more time to recover. That could lead to better results, or it could just be a more enjoyable way to work out.

It's also possible that total-body workouts are simply too difficult. You have to focus, by necessity, on exercises like squats and presses, which use your body's biggest and strongest muscles in coordinated movements. It might be too much fatigue for one workout, in which case it makes more sense to spread the work across 4 days instead of 3, assuming your schedule allows it.

There's no evidence that one is better than the other. A friend of mine, Brad Schoenfeld, PhD, does a lot of research into the nuances of muscle building. His studies show that the total amount of work is the most important factor. Whether you train each muscle group two or three times a week shouldn't matter as much as the quality and quantity of that work.

Specific to someone with diabetes, I see two possible benefits to split routines.

- First, and most obvious, it's one more workout a week. That's one more opportunity to get up and move, to make your muscles work, and to improve your body's strength and functional abilities.

- Second, it gives you an opportunity to do more exercise *in addition* to strength training. For example, if you're in a gym anyway, you might do 15 to 20 minutes of cardio exercise before or after lifting. At home you might do more stretches or mobility exercises. You might do more stability training for your core muscles. Even if none of that additional exercise is especially strenuous or fatiguing, it's still more than you would've done with fewer workouts.

## THE PROGRAM

Here's what you'll do in each workout.

## WORKOUT 1

| EXERCISE | SETS | REPS |
| --- | --- | --- |
| Chest press | 3 | 8–12 |
| Row | 3 | 8–12 |
| Shoulder press | 3 | 8–12 |
| Biceps curl | 2–3 | 8–12 |
| Triceps extension (optional) | 2–3 | 8–12 |
| Pushup hold | 2–3 | 30–60 seconds |

# WORKOUT 2

| EXERCISE | SETS | REPS |
|---|---|---|
| Squat | 3 | 8–12 |
| Split squat | 3 | 8–12* |
| Stiff-legged deadlift or leg curl | 3 | 8–12 |
| Hip raise (strength) | 3 | 8–12 |
| Curlup | 2–3 | 4–6† |

*Each leg

†Hold each contraction for up to 10 seconds.

# WORKOUT 3

| EXERCISE | SETS | REPS |
|---|---|---|
| Incline chest press | 4 | 6–8 |
| Lat pulldown or inverted row | 4 | 6–8 |
| Shrug | 4 | 6–8 |
| Upright row or lateral raise | 4 | 6–8 |
| Bird dog | 1–2 | 60 seconds* |
| Side bridge | 1–2 | 3–4†‡ |

*Hold each position for 10 seconds, then switch sides, and continue for just over 1 minute per set.

†Each side

‡Hold for up to 10 seconds at a time, relax, and repeat, for a total time of at least 30 seconds per side on each set.

# WORKOUT 4

| EXERCISE | SETS | REPS |
|---|---|---|
| Deadlift | 4 | 6–8 |
| Front squat or leg press | 4 | 6–8 |
| Stepup | 4 | 6–8* |
| Hip raise (stability) | 2–3 | 30–60 seconds† |
| Plank | 2–3 | 30–60 seconds† |

*Each leg

†Hold for up to 10 seconds at a time, relax, and repeat, for a total time of 30 to 60 seconds per set.

# HOW TO DO THE PROGRAM

**Workouts:** You'll get the best results if you do each workout once a week, with no more than two workouts on consecutive days. An ideal schedule would be:

| | |
|---|---|
| Monday | Workout 1 |
| Tuesday | Workout 2 |
| Thursday | Workout 3 |
| Friday | Workout 4 |

**Warmup sets:** I recommend a warmup set for the first exercise in each workout. You probably want to use between 50 and 75 percent of the weight you'd select for a normal set of that exercise, and do 8 to 10 reps. The purpose of the warmup set is to practice the movement without exhausting your muscles.

**Weight selection:** You'll do 8 to 12 reps per set in Workout 1 and Workout 2, and 6 to 8 reps in Workout 3 and Workout 4. The goal is the same: to fatigue your muscles. So when you're doing higher reps, by the time you get to the 10th or 11th rep, it should feel as if you can *maybe* do one or two more, but there's a risk you wouldn't be able to do them with good form. (When the last one or two reps are noticeably slower than the previous ones, that's usually a good time to stop the set.)

It works the same way when you're doing six to eight reps. You want your muscles to feel pretty tired by the sixth or seventh repetition. Because you're doing fewer reps, you'll need to use heavier weights to reach that level of fatigue.

In any workout, you need to increase the weight when you reach the top of the range—the 8th or 12th repetition—and feel as if you could do more without compromising your form.

**Rest:** There's no fixed amount of time you need for recovery between sets. It might be 30 seconds when doing higher reps with lighter weights, and up to 60 seconds when you're working with heavier weights for fewer reps. The only rule: If you don't need *any* rest, you didn't use nearly enough weight on that set.

# EXERCISES

I covered the basic versions of most of these exercises in Chapter 12, and then added "gym options" for those who work out in a commercial health club. Here I'll describe a few more variations, including several with a barbell.

Ordinarily I wouldn't recommend using a barbell unless you're an experienced lifter with ambitious goals for building strength and/or muscle size. But many of you may already have a barbell set, or know someone who has one sitting around unused and would be happy to get rid of it. Whether you do or don't, the barbell may be the most practical equipment option for a reasonably strong man or woman who works out at home. It's less expensive than a complete range of dumbbells, or a set of selectorized dumbbells heavy enough for a stronger-than-average lifter. A barbell also allows you to do inverted rows and deadlifts at home, two exercises that would otherwise be impractical, if not impossible. Finally, the plates themselves have multiple uses, as you'll see.

However, if you're going to use a barbell, you'll also need some kind of rack to raise it up off the floor for squats, inverted rows, and chest presses. Your best options are adjustable squat stands or a one-piece workout rack with supports that you can adjust up or down for different exercises. You should be able to get either one online for less than $100 at Amazon or Jet.com; at brick-and-mortar sporting goods stores; or at the Web sites for big-box retailers like Walmart or Sears.

# Exercises in Workout 1

Everything shown or described in Chapter 12—pushup variations, dumbbells, machines—is still an option in this program.

## BARBELL CHEST PRESS

Lie on your back on the bench with the barbell positioned on the supports just slightly below arm's length. Make sure the back of your head, upper back, and glutes rest on the bench, with a slight arch in your lower back. Spread your feet wide. Grab the bar overhand, with your hands just beyond shoulder-width apart, and lift it off the supports. Hold it directly over your chest. That's the starting position. Bend your elbows and lower the bar to your chest. Pause, and then push it back to the starting position.

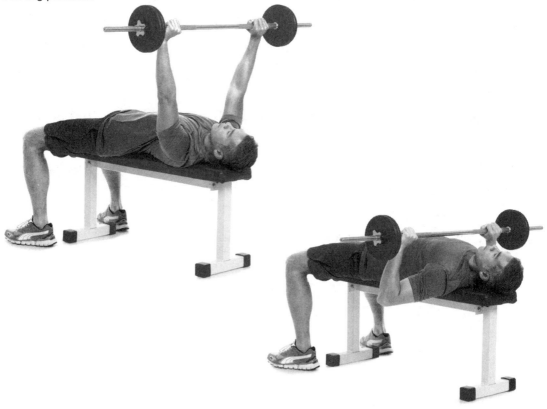

## ROW

Again, every option from the last chapter is open to you: dumbbell, resistance band, cable, machines. So is the barbell, which as I said can be pretty tough on your lower back. But if it's your best (or only) option, the barbell bent-over row can be a good exercise. You just need to be careful with form and avoid positions that strain your back.

### BARBELL BENT-OVER ROW

Grab the bar overhand with your hands just beyond shoulder width. Stand with your feet about shoulder-width apart. Bend forward at the hips so your torso is at a 45-degree angle to the floor, with your arms hanging straight down from your shoulders and perpendicular to the floor, and your knees bent. Tighten everything from your shoulders through your hips. Pull the bar straight up to your abdomen, pause, and lower it back to the starting position.

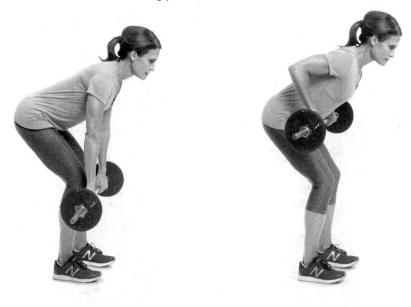

### Variation

You can also use an underhand grip, with your hands a bit closer together, to give more work to your biceps.

## SHOULDER PRESS

The dumbbell versions from the previous chapter are still your best choices here. The barbell press is harder to learn and easier to mess up. But like the barbell row, it can be a productive exercise if you pay careful attention to your form. Stop your set if you feel a strain in one or both shoulders, or in your lower back. That applies to both the dumbbell and barbell versions.

### BARBELL SHOULDER PRESS

If you have supports, raise them to about chest level, and set the barbell in them. If not, you'll have to pick the bar up from the floor. Either way, grab the bar overhand with your hands about shoulder-width apart. Lift it off the supports or lift it from the floor, and hold it in front of your shoulders with your elbows pushed slightly forward. (Put another way, you *don't* want your elbows directly below your hands, with your forearms perpendicular to the floor.) Push the bar up and back slightly, tilting your head back to get your chin out of the way, until your arms are straight and the bar is directly over the top of your head. Lower it along the same path, again moving your head back.

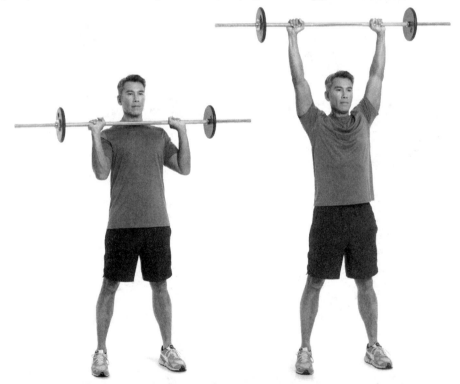

## BICEPS CURL

Use any of the variations from Chapter 12.

# TRICEPS EXTENSION (OPTIONAL)

This is an optional exercise because your triceps already get a lot of work with the two pressing movements. (Your biceps, by contrast, would get used only in the row if I didn't include the curl in the workout.) Most people who work out in gyms prefer to work their triceps with the cable machine that's designed for it. You just set the bar at chest level, grab it with both hands a few inches in front of your torso, and straighten your arms. With good form you also get a bit of work for your core. At home, your best option is the dumbbell extension shown here. You can also use a barbell, but it can be very tough on your elbows.

## DUMBBELL TRICEPS EXTENSION

Grab a pair of light dumbbells and lie on your back on the bench, holding them directly over your chest like you're going to do a chest press. Now turn your palms in toward each other, and shift your arms back toward your head slightly, so they're no longer perpendicular to your torso. That's the starting position. Without moving your upper arms, bend your elbows until the weights are alongside your head, just behind your ears. Straighten your arms to return to the starting position.

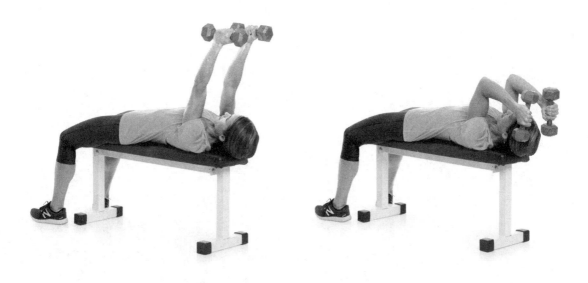

## Variation

You can also do standing extensions, using one or two dumbbells. If you use one, hold one end with both hands, and lower it behind your head.

# PUSHUP HOLD

This stability exercise is as simple as it gets: Get into pushup position, with your hands about shoulder-width apart and your weight supported on your hands and toes. Set your body in a straight line from neck to ankles, and hold for 30 to 60 seconds. Keep your entire body tight, paying special attention to your lower back and pelvis. Ideally, your posture in the pushup position is the same as it would be if you were standing up with your arms out in front of your chest.

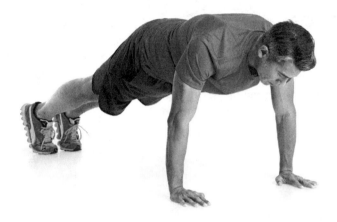

## Variations

- Need a bigger challenge? You can set your feet on a step or bench. (This angle might actually be easier on your back, even if it's tougher for your core muscles.)

- An even bigger challenge: Set your feet on something unstable, like an inflatable exercise ball, or in the straps of a suspension system. (Just make sure the suspension device is attached to something sturdy, like a ceiling joist in your garage or a chinup bar in your gym.)

- Need to dial it back? Do the pushup hold with your hands elevated on a step or bench.

# Exercises in Workout 2

## SQUAT

The goblet squat I described in Chapter 12 is the very best option for most novice to intermediate lifters. But as you get stronger, it's harder to manage. Men especially can quickly outgrow the maximum weight of the dumbbells at home, a community fitness center, or even a commercial gym like Planet Fitness. Buying single dumbbells in 5- or 10-pound increments gets expensive (up to $1 a pound). Then there's the problem of where to put them in between workouts. That's when the barbell squat becomes a more appealing option, even though it's an exercise that takes some time to master.

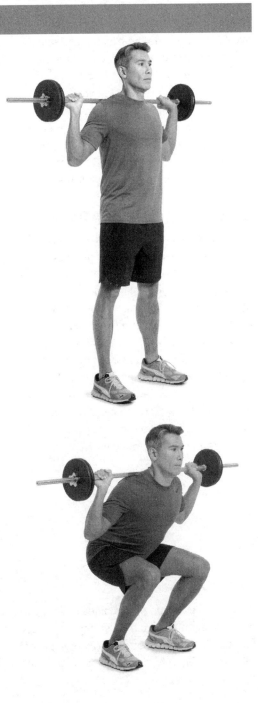

### BARBELL BACK SQUAT

Set the bar on the supports at chest height. Grab the bar with your hands as wide as they need to be for comfort. Duck under the bar and brace it against your upper back, just below your neck. Squeeze your shoulder blades together so it has a cushion to rest on. Lift it off the supports and step back, setting your feet about shoulder-width apart and your toes forward, or turned out slightly.

Now push your hips back and descend as far you can, keeping your heels on the floor, your head up, and your chest pointed forward. Make sure your knees stay aligned with your toes—don't let them collapse inward. Lift back up to the starting position.

### SPLIT SQUAT

You can do any variation shown in the previous chapter.

## STIFF-LEGGED DEADLIFT OR LEG CURL

The deadlift is a key strength exercise. You'll see two versions in this program: In Workout 4 you'll do the traditional deadlift, in which you start with the weight near the floor; and here in Workout 2 you'll do the stiff-legged deadlift, in which you hold the weight in front of your torso and lower it toward the floor. The former is more of a total-body exercise, while this one more directly works your glutes and hamstrings (the muscles on the back of your thighs).

### STIFF-LEGGED DEADLIFT

You can do this exercise with a barbell or pair of dumbbells. Whichever you choose, stand holding the weights with straight arms in front of your thighs. Set your feet about shoulder-width apart, toes forward. Push your hips back and lower the weights toward the floor, keeping your back straight and your shoulders and torso tight. Stop when the weights are just below your knees, or sooner if you feel your lower back start to shift out of its natural arch. Push your hips forward and return to the starting position.

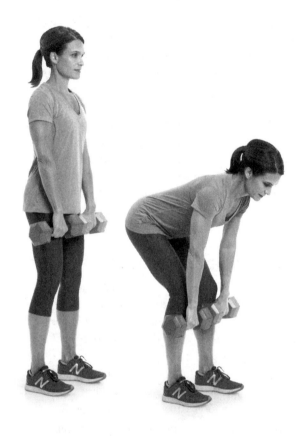

### LEG CURL

If you have a choice of machines in your gym, you can use either one: lying or seated. They're both pretty straightforward: Adjust the ankle support and/or seat (ask a gym employee to help you the first time), and then bend your knees against the resistance the machine provides. You should feel this almost entirely in your hamstrings, with some work for your calves.

## HIP RAISE

As with the deadlift, there are two versions of the hip raise in this program. Here in Workout 2 you'll do it as described in the previous chapter. Since you'll probably need to use a weight, I'll explain how to do it with a barbell. In Workout 4 you'll use just your body weight or a mini-band, and then hold the top position for time.

### BARBELL HIP RAISE

Sit on the floor with your legs straight. Roll the barbell up your legs until it reaches your lap. Or, if you can't roll it up, lift one end and slide underneath it, with the middle of the bar over your hips. Hold it in place with both hands and lie on your back. Bend your knees and set your feet shoulder-width apart and flat on the floor. This is your starting position. Push your hips up so your body forms a straight line from chest to knees. Pause, then lower your hips back to the floor. If it's uncomfortable to support the bar on your lap, wrap a towel around it, or put a rubber pad between the bar and your pelvis.

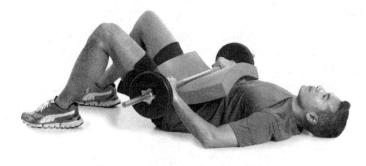

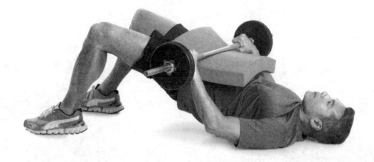

## CURLUP

Use it as described in Chapter 12.

# Exercises in Workout 3

## LAT PULLDOWN OR INVERTED ROW

Humans are built to climb, with relatively long arms, strong upper-back muscles, and shoulder joints that allow an extreme range of motion. But modern life makes it really hard to mimic that climbing motion and to fully employ those muscles. Even in the gym, it isn't easy—or at least it wasn't, when chinups, pullups, and rope climbing were the only options. The invention of the lat pulldown machine changed that. Now anyone can work the same muscles used for climbing, even if he or she isn't nearly strong enough to do a chinup.

Alas, it's rarely an option for those who work out at home. The next-best solution is the inverted row. It allows you to work the same muscles you'd use in a pulldown, only without having to lift your entire body weight.

### INVERTED ROW

Set a barbell in the supports at about hip height. Position yourself under the bar. You can grasp it overhand, with your hands just outside shoulder width, or underhand, with your hands a bit closer together. Hang from the bar and set your body in a straight line from neck to ankles, with your weight resting on your heels. Pull your chest up to the bar. If that's too challenging, you can either raise the bar, or bend your knees and move your feet up closer. Whatever position you end up in, you should be able to do at least 6 reps per set, but no more than 10.

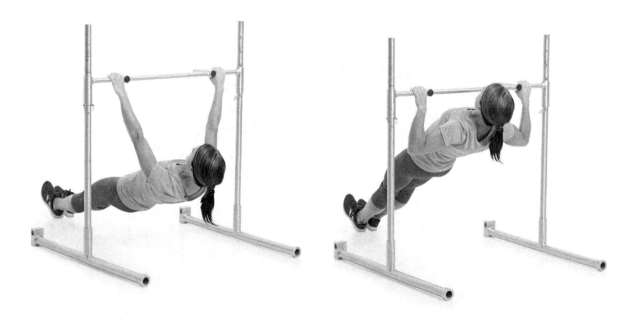

## INVERTED ROW OPTION: SUSPENDED ROW

If you belong to a gym, you'll probably see a suspension system (TRX is the best-known brand) hanging from a chinup bar. It's a great choice for inverted rows. To get in the starting position, you grab the handles, walk out until the straps and your arms are both fully extended, and then walk your heels back in until your body is diagonal to the floor. From there you just pull the handles to your sides. As before, you want to find an angle that allows you to hit the minimum number of reps over four sets.

## LAT PULLDOWN

Attach a long bar to the overhead pulley, and adjust the machine's seat and knee support to fit your dimensions. Grab the bar overhand with a grip that's somewhat wider than your shoulders. Position yourself on the seat, with your knees beneath the support pad. Lean back slightly and tighten your arms, shoulders, and back. Pull the bar to your upper chest, pause, and extend your arms back to the starting position.

## LAT PULLDOWN OPTIONS

If your gym has dual handles, you can use those instead of a straight bar. You can also use the straight bar with an underhand grip, or try some of the other attachments your gym makes available. The key to any variation is to pull the bar down to your *chest,* not to your stomach or your lap. You should feel your upper-back muscles squeeze when the bar or handles reach your chest.

## INCLINE CHEST PRESS

As described in the last chapter, you can do this with dumbbells or a barbell. Set the bench to whatever incline is comfortable for you—probably 30 to 45 degrees.

# SHRUG

Your shoulder blades have several important functions. They move away from each other when you reach forward, rotate out and up when you reach overhead, and do the opposite movements when you pull something toward your body. Good posture requires them to stay down and tight, but they also need to be able to move straight up, as when you shrug your shoulders. These actions all happen without your having to give them any thought; they're just a normal part of lifting, throwing, climbing, cleaning, or anything else you do with your arms and shoulders.

But when you have a mostly sedentary life, especially if you do a lot of typing or driving, a strange thing happens: Your shoulder blades stop moving as smoothly as they should. A good strength-training program will include exercises that get the shoulder blades working again. The pushup, for example, uses muscles that pull them apart, while rowing exercises bring them together. The shoulder press makes them rotate out and lift up; the lat pulldown, as its name suggests, has them rotate in and pull down.

The shrug is another whose name tells you exactly what the goal is. But it's unique in that it's the only exercise in my program that has no purpose other than working the upper-back muscles responsible for elevating your shoulder blades. Well, okay, there's one more benefit: If you are fairly strong and use reasonably heavy weights, you'll also improve your grip strength.

## BARBELL OR DUMBBELL SHRUG

Hold a barbell in front of your thighs or a pair of dumbbells at your sides. Shrug your shoulders up toward your ears, pause for a moment to feel the squeeze in your upper-back muscles, and lower the weight.

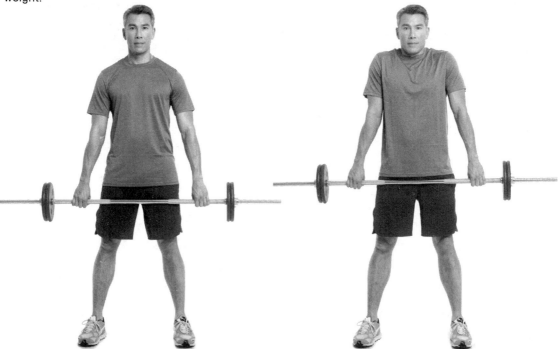

# UPRIGHT ROW OR LATERAL RAISE

These exercises directly work the muscles on the outsides of your shoulders.

## UPRIGHT ROW

Hold a barbell or pair of dumbbells in front of your thighs. Lift the weights straight up your torso until your upper arms are parallel to the floor. Don't go any higher; that can lead to shoulder problems. Pause to feel the squeeze across your shoulders and upper back, then lower the weights to the starting position.

## LATERAL RAISE

Hold a pair of light dumbbells at your sides, with your hands turned toward each other and elbows bent slightly. Lift your arms straight out to your sides until they're parallel to the floor. Pause and lower them to the starting position. You can also do this exercise with a pair of weight plates instead of dumbbells.

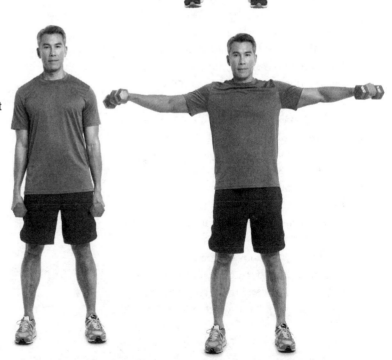

# BIRD DOG AND SIDE BRIDGE

These are the same as in Chapter 12.

# Exercises in Workout 4

## DEADLIFT

I mentioned a moment ago that the deadlift is a total-body exercise. It works the small gripping muscles in your hands and forearms; the large upper-back muscles that hold your arms and shoulders in place and make lifting heavy objects possible; the absolutely crucial core muscles that keep your lower back and pelvis locked in a safe, stable position; and of course the big, strong muscles in your hips and thighs, the ones that actually lift the weight off the floor.

It's also perhaps the most practical exercise in this or any strength program you'll find. As my friends in the fitness industry like to say, heavy things don't lift themselves. That's equally true of groceries, sofas, luggage, and sleeping children.

### DUMBBELL OR KETTLEBELL DEADLIFT

You can do this with a barbell, dumbbell, or kettlebell. If you have a choice, I recommend using either of the latter choices. Stand over the weight with your feet wide apart and toes turned out slightly. (If you're using a dumbbell, stand it upright.) Push your hips back, bend your knees, reach down, and grab the top or handle with both hands. Pull your shoulders down, stick your chest out, and tighten everything from your hands to your feet. Your arms should be straight, your head up, and your eyes focused straight ahead. Now push your hips forward and straighten your body as you pull the weight off the floor. Lower it all the way to the floor and reset your body before starting the next repetition.

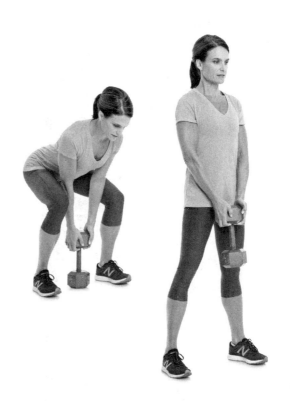

## BARBELL DEADLIFT

This variation allows you to work with heavier weights, if you need to, but is also riskier for your back. You have to be extremely careful to keep your shoulders, core, and hips tight; they should be like a single unit when they move. One other precaution: If possible, you want the starting position of the bar to be about the same height as the dumbbell or kettlebell I just described—8 to 10 inches above the floor. If you have, and can use, weight plates that are 17 to 18 inches in diameter, you'll be fine. With smaller plates, you may want to elevate the bar. You can place a couple of weight plates on the floor and roll the bar up onto them, or set the bar on a pair of low boxes, boards, or steps.

Once your bar is ready, set your feet shoulder-width apart, with your shins touching the bar. Grab the bar overhand, with your hands just outside your legs and about shoulder-width apart. Straighten your arms, pull down your shoulders, push out your chest, fix your eyes on a spot straight ahead, tighten everything, and pull the bar straight up your shins to your mid-thighs. Lower it to the floor and reset your body before lifting again.

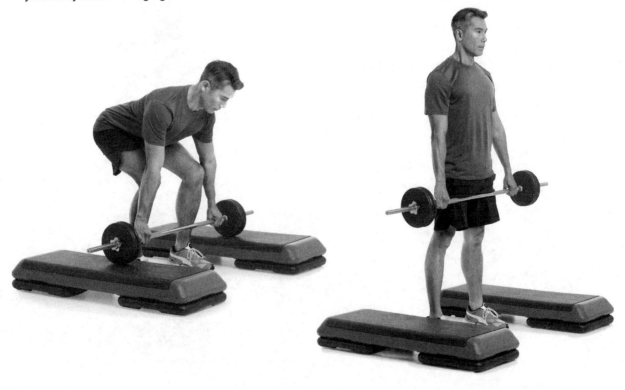

# FRONT SQUAT OR LEG PRESS

The goal with a front squat is to work the same muscles as the back squat I described for Workout 2, but with your torso more upright. So if you work out at home with a barbell, your best option here in Workout 4 is the barbell front squat.

If you planned to use the goblet squat in Workout 2, doing a front squat in this workout is redundant. The goblet squat already forces you to keep your torso upright. You have two options: In a fully equipped gym, the leg press is an easy choice. At home with dumbbells, you can try the dumbbell front squat.

## BARBELL FRONT SQUAT

Set the barbell in the supports at about chest height. Grab the bar overhand, with your hands just outside your shoulders. Rotate your arms under and around the bar until your elbows point forward and your palms are turned toward the ceiling. The bar should sit on your front shoulders, up against your collarbone. As long as you keep your elbows up, it'll stay there.

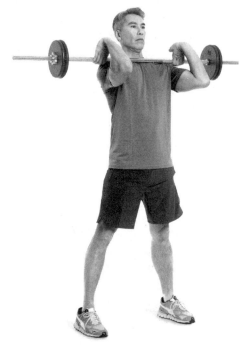

Lift the bar off the supports and step back. Set your feet shoulder-width apart, with your toes pointed forward or turned out a bit, whichever is more comfortable. Tighten your shoulders and torso. Push your hips back and lower yourself as far as you can while keeping your lower back in its naturally arched position. Lift yourself back up to the starting position.

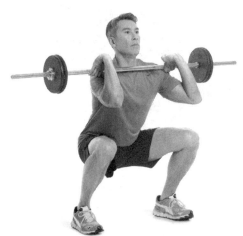

## LEG PRESS

You'll probably need a gym employee to show you how to set up the machine and adjust the seat. You may also need to load weight plates onto the machine. (Don't be timid with the weights; the way some of these machines are engineered, what seems like a huge load can be entirely manageable and even necessary for a good workout.) Once you're set up, just put your feet on the platform about shoulder-width apart, brace your back on the pad, and push the weight until your legs are fully extended. Be careful on the return; you need to keep it under control so you don't lift your hips off the pad and shift the load to your lower back.

## DUMBBELL FRONT SQUAT

Take two dumbbells and flip them up onto the meaty parts of your shoulders. Your elbows will point forward with your palms turned toward your ears. Do the squat as described opposite.

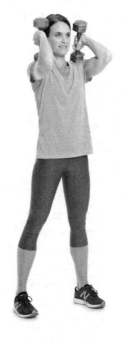

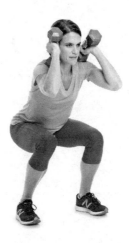

# STEPUP

This is a simple exercise that works your leg muscles the way they would be used if you were climbing stairs. In other words, it strengthens the muscles through a movement pattern that you've probably used every day since you learned to walk, and hope to use for many years in the future.

At first you may not need to use any weight at all. The heavier you are, the more challenging it will be. If you need to use a load, you have a world of options. The simplest is to hold a dumbbell in each hand, as shown below. You can also use kettlebells, a barbell, or a single weight plate held against your chest. You can hold weights at your side, at your shoulders, or even overhead.

Whatever option you choose, you'll need a box or step that's sturdy enough to hold your weight. Most people will do well with a box that's 12 to 18 inches high. But if you're heavier, shorter, or have knee issues, a lower box is fine.

## DUMBBELL STEPUP

Grab a pair of dumbbells and stand with your left foot flat on the step and your right foot on the floor. Push through your heel and lift your body up so your right foot is even with your left. Lower your right foot to the floor and repeat, doing all your reps with your left leg before you repeat with your right foot on the step. Make sure the top leg does all the work; the trailing leg is just along for the ride.

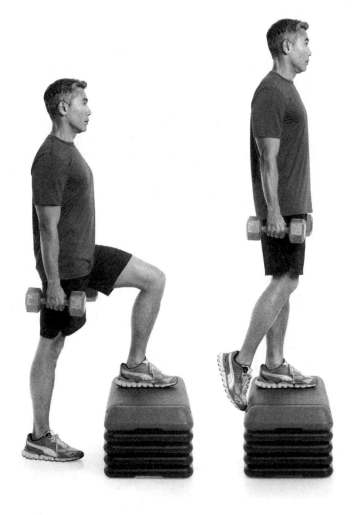

## HIP RAISE

In Workout 4, you'll do the hip raise as a stability exercise, rather than to build strength. Your goal is to develop endurance in your hip muscles. So you'll get into the "up" position—with your body straight from chest to knees—and hold for up to 10 seconds at a time before you lower your hips and repeat. Do three to six reps per set, or 30 to 60 seconds altogether. If that's not challenging enough, wear a mini-band around your thighs. That forces you to push your knees out at the same time you're lifting your hips up, essentially doubling the benefits of the exercise.

## PLANK

This is exactly like the pushup hold from Workout 1, except you're balancing your weight on your forearms and toes. Use the same holding pattern I described for the hip raise: Hold for up to 10 seconds, lower yourself, and repeat, aiming for 30 to 60 seconds per set.

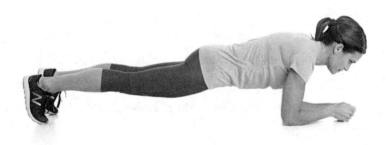

# A Few More Words of Caution

I explained in Chapter 4 why it's so important to get your doctor's input before beginning an exercise program. When ramping up a program, your goal is to avoid creating problems that will send you back to the doctor. The toughest injuries are those that arise from successful workouts. Your muscles and joints adapt to training asymmetrically. Because your muscles have a richer blood supply, they're much better at building and repairing themselves. Your connective tissues, with less bloodflow, will lag behind. So if your strength or endurance increases rapidly, it's entirely possible, and even predictable, that at some point you'll strain or inflame tendons or ligaments, or damage cartilage in your knees or shoulders.

Most of the time, your body gives you warning signs in the early stages of an overuse injury. A lifter or swimmer might experience discomfort in one or both of his shoulders. A runner or lifter might have knee pain that lasts for a day or two after a long run or heavy workout. Lifters, golfers, and tennis players can develop chronic elbow soreness.

What to do?

1. **If it hurts *while* you're doing it, stop.** Like, *immediately.* You can try another variation of the exercise, or try it at a slower pace, or you can just call it a day and see what happens.

2. **If it hurts after you do it, take an extra day or two to recover.** Then reassess, doing a lighter, slower, or more cautious version of the workout. If

post-workout soreness is entirely in the muscle, it means you pushed yourself a bit harder than usual or hit your body with an unfamiliar challenge. It's the price you sometimes pay for being ambitious. But if it's all or mostly in a joint, you need to be very, very careful about how hard you push it in the next few days or weeks.

3. **Stay within the pain-free range of motion.** This rule applies to all training, but it's especially urgent when you're returning from an injury. No matter what the exercise instructions say, or how you see an exercise performed in a video, you never want to do an exercise in a way that causes pain, and you'll pay a steep price if you try. It's possible to increase your pain-free range of motion over time, with careful practice and increasing skill. But you can't rush the process.

4. **If pain persists, get it checked out.** See a doctor or physical therapist, or at least ask a trainer or rehab professional for some guidance. There may be a better way to do the exercise or activity, or alternative exercises you can try, or something completely different that still helps you reach your goals. Just remember that pain is your body's way of saying you have a problem that needs to be fixed or worked around, and to continue what you've been doing will only make it worse.

# PART FOUR

# TREATMENT AND RECOVERY

## CHAPTER 14

# The Power, Peril, and Limits of Diabetes Medications

**REMEMBER THAT FACTORY I TALKED ABOUT** in Chapter 2, and briefly revisited in Chapter 8? The one with the cargo piling up on the loading docks because the doors stopped opening with the press of a button? Picture yourself working there. Whatever you do in real life—accounting, sales, management, landscaping—that's what you do at the factory. One day your boss comes up to you and says, "Things are really going pear-shaped here, and we all have to work harder until we get back on track. And to show you how much I appreciate what you're about to do, I'm going to provide the extra coffee you'll need to power through it."

You're a team player, right? So you drink the coffee, work the longer hours, and get the job done . . . for a while. Then your productivity falls off. You feel like you're only half awake during those long daytime hours, but only half asleep at night, thanks to the caffeine.

It's not long before your boss notices. "I'm sorry," you tell him. "My system can't handle this constant stress."

But instead of cutting your hours, or decreasing your workload, your boss hands you a bottle of amphetamines. "Start with one a day," he tells you. "If that isn't enough, you can take two."

"And what if *that* doesn't work?" you ask, your voice quavering with anger and incredulity. "Should I take three? How about four?"

"No, of course not!" he answers, not picking up on your sarcasm. "That would be crazy! If a double dose isn't enough, we'll just find another drug. There's *always* another one to try." He says this in his most reassuring voice as he ushers you out of his office and his assistant leads the next half-asleep employee in.

I'm sure you've guessed the point of this little parable, and it's not to give you flashbacks to that job where your boss really would've given you speed if he thought he could get away with it. (Or to remind me of my final year of med school.) It's to reiterate a point I made earlier: Type 2 diabetes is a disease of excess—too much food, and too much time sitting still instead of moving around. The answer to an excess of nutrition should not be an excess of medicine.

Those drugs, separately and in various combinations, certainly lower blood glucose, at least temporarily. But each year, 5 to 10 percent of patients taking just one medication fail to keep their hemoglobin A1C below the target level. Within 3 years, 50 percent need a second one. And after 9 years, 75 percent of patients are using multiple drugs.

We call that polypharmacy, and our patients may take those drugs along with others prescribed for high blood pressure, depression, or any of the other conditions we often see tag-teaming with diabetes and obesity. My goal, both in my practice and in these pages, is to help you keep those prescriptions to an absolute minimum. It's hardly original for me to point out that medicine, no matter how powerful, can only address symptoms. And even the safest ones come with a risk of side effects, which in some cases require additional medications to treat. If it's possible to address the *cause* of diabetes, we owe it to ourselves to do exactly that.

# DRUG BUST

I'm an American doctor, writing a book for an American publisher, which means most of you readers also live in the United States, where drug prices are just nuts. I understand that companies spend fantastic sums to research and develop new drugs, and I don't have any philosophical problem with them turning a profit. But I also see them spend fantastic sums on marketing and advertising, and I know that much of their research goes into "me too" drugs, which are designed to compete with similar products from other companies, and in most cases won't work any better. They may actually be worse.

Similarly, the price of generic drugs makes absolutely no sense. Due to consolidation, fewer companies make more drugs, leading to unpredictable shortages and random price changes.

Insurance companies pass more of these price increases on to their customers. On top of that, many of my patients change insurance policies every year—moving from one provider to another, or to different plans offered by the same company. That means new rules every 12 months, with potentially dramatic shifts in which drugs are covered and how much of the sticker price they'll have to pay.

All this frustrates the hell out of everybody. My patients often don't know what their drugs will cost from one month to the next, never mind what they might have to pay next year. I can't always prescribe the medications I think are best for my patients because of the prohibitive price tag. Even insurance companies, whose profits depend on their customers staying healthy, don't know which of the newer ones are worth the high cost, and which are just expensive replacements for older, cheaper, and equally effective drugs.

So keep in mind, as I describe the most effective drugs, that some of them may not be covered by your insurance, or may be unaffordable even if they are.

So when I talk about drugs in this chapter and the next, it's with the understanding that they work best as adjuncts to everything we've talked about in the preceding chapters—nutrition, weight management, exercise, and better sleep.

## METFORMIN

You know by now that eating a meal, especially one high in carbohydrates, leads to a quick rise in blood sugar. It's entirely normal, and usually transient. You also know that someone with diabetes has chronically elevated blood glucose. In part it's because your cells become insensitive to insulin, and like the doors on the loading docks of that dysfunctional factory, they can't open up and take the glucose out of your blood. But it's also because your liver makes too much glucose from other materials, like amino acids and triglycerides, through a process called *hepatic gluconeogenesis.* It then sends that glucose into your bloodstream, where it only makes things worse.

Metformin somehow blocks this process, and by preventing some of that new glucose from forming, it lowers your blood sugar. I say "somehow" because it's been studied off and on for nearly a century, and we still aren't completely sure how it works. Scientists discovered back in the 1920s that chemicals found in a plant called goat's rue, or French lilac, lowered blood sugar in animals. But by then doctors had insulin to treat people with diabetes, and no one followed up on their discovery until the 1950s. Even then the rollout was slow; metformin wasn't approved in the United States for type 2 diabetes until 1994.

Today metformin is the most commonly used diabetes drug in the world, and the first one I prescribe for patients with elevated A1C, including those with prediabetes. It's cheap and effective, and it has relatively few side effects. Those are generally limited to flatulence, but can include nausea, cramping, and diarrhea. I also see modest weight loss in some of my patients, although it's nothing close to what they achieve with diet and exercise.

The more research we have, the better metformin looks. We know it lowers triglycerides and LDL particles, and may have promising applications in cancer treatment. There's even been some buzz about metformin as a potential anti-aging drug. But for diabetes, it's the first medicine I prescribe, and in most cases I hope it's also the last.

## BEYOND METFORMIN

If a patient comes into my office with an A1C that's 7.5 or higher, or if metformin alone doesn't bring A1C down to the target level (which will vary, depending on the individual), my next step is to try metformin in combination with one of these.

**GLP-1 agonists.** Glucagon-like peptide 1 is a hormone produced by your intestines that stimulates insulin release. At the same time, it puts the brakes on glucagon, a hormone that does the opposite of insulin by *raising* your blood sugar when it falls too low—a crucial function when there isn't enough glucose in your blood to supply your brain. So if it's been a few hours since your last meal, glucagon tells your liver to convert some of its glycogen back into glucose, or to create glucose from other nutrients, as I described a moment ago.

With diabetes, your body produces less GLP-1, leaving you with dangerously high levels of blood sugar. A GLP-1 agonist is an injectable drug that targets the same receptors. So even though it's a synthetic version of the hormone, your body responds as it would to the real thing. (The opposite would be an antagonist that blocks a hormone's actions.) In addition to blunting glucagon release, GLP-1 also makes you less hungry through a pair of complementary mechanisms: It weakens hunger signals coming from the brain, and also increases post-meal satiety by slowing down the transit of food from your digestive system into your bloodstream.

The one I use most often is liraglutide, sold under the brand name Victoza, a name you would probably recognize from TV commercials even if you didn't have diabetes. It's associated with more weight loss than other drugs in this category, but also requires daily injections, which is a deal breaker for many of my patients. For them I generally turn to dulaglutide (Trulicity), which is injected once a week.

**SGLT2 inhibitors.** Sodium-glucose cotransporter 2 sounds like the worst movie of Jason Statham's career. But despite the long name, these proteins do something fairly simple: They allow glucose to be reabsorbed from your kidneys and sent back into your bloodstream. An SGLT2 inhibitor prevents that reabsorption, allowing you to get rid of excess glucose through your urine. Your blood sugar goes down, you lose weight (you're literally pissing away calories), and your blood pressure declines as well. I've used three medicines in this class with good results: canagliflozin (Invokana), dapagliflozin (Farxiga), and empagliflozin (Jardiance). The latter was linked to a significantly lower risk of death from heart disease in a recent study.

**DPP-4 inhibitors.** For patients who don't want to use the injectable GLP-1 inhibitors, I sometimes prescribe one of these medicines. They block an enzyme called dipeptidyl peptidase-4, which breaks down GLP-1. This results in your body having more of your natural GLP-1, leading to lower blood sugar and better satiety between meals. DPP-4 inhibitors are mostly weight neutral—that is, not associated with weight loss or gain. Drugs in this category include sitagliptin (Januvia), linagliptin (Tradjenta), saxagliptin (Onglyza), and alogliptin (Nesina).

**TZDs.** Thiazolidinediones aren't just hard to pronounce; they also have some scary side effects, including weight gain, an increased risk of bone fractures, and chronic edema (holding excess water in your extremities). But the weight gain isn't entirely bad; you're less likely to store visceral fat around your middle and more likely to store subcutaneous fat around your hips and thighs. On the plus side, they're the only blood-sugar-lowering drugs known to reduce insulin resistance directly. Pioglitazone (Actos), the only drug in this class that I currently prescribe, may also offer a mild cardiovascular benefit.

**Drugs I rarely use.** Acarbose (Precose) and miglitol (Glyset) prevent the breakdown of starches. When fewer carbs get into your bloodstream, your blood sugar goes down. But those carbs don't give up without a fight. Almost everyone in Western countries who uses acarbose gets mild to severe flatulence, and many also get diarrhea. But Asians, who typically have more of the enzymes that break down starch, due to a traditionally grain-heavy diet, tolerate these drugs much better than those whose ancestors came from Europe, Africa, or the Americas. I use them successfully with Asian American patients who are prediabetic and don't want to stop eating rice with most meals.

Colesevelam (Welchol) blocks the absorption of fats, which explains why it was originally used to lower LDL. It also lowers blood sugar, although not by much, and has a neutral effect on body weight. Side effects include constipation. I haven't used it with many patients.

Bromocriptine (Cycloset) is a psychoactive drug that stimulates the release of dopamine. It's been used to treat Parkinson's disease (which kills the cells in the brain that manufacture dopamine) as well as cocaine addiction (which stimulates the reward system, including dopamine receptors). Bromocriptine lowers blood sugar a bit and may also have cardiovascular benefits, but it's not a drug I've ever used with my patients. I leave the psychoactive drugs to those who specialize in them.

**SFUs: my least favorite drug of all.** There's another meaning of SFU (usually with a "t" between the S and F), which pretty accurately describes my reaction when I see this class of drugs recommended by my fellow doctors. Sulfonylureas act like a turbocharger to get your pancreas to squeeze out more insulin. They bring your blood glucose down quickly and cheaply, but sometimes it comes down so far that you end up with hypoglycemia—low blood sugar. They also lead to weight gain, thanks to the insulin forcing more nutrients into your cells. These drugs, in effect, take an excess of energy intake and turn it into an excess of energy storage, creating a new problem without addressing the original one.

I mention this class of drugs—which includes glyburide (DiaBeta), glipizide (Glucotrol), glimepiride (Amaryl), and nateglinide (Starlix)—only because they're still listed near the top of the treatment recommendations we use, right after metformin. And like metformin, they're certainly affordable. I don't prescribe them unless I can't avoid it, and if a new patient is already using them, I try to switch him to something else.

# INSULIN

Insulin is the most powerful drug I can prescribe for type 2 diabetes. It's also the one I'm most reluctant to use, unless I think the patient's health is in imminent danger. That's because patients often gain weight with insulin. To understand why, let's quickly review what this hormone is and what it does.

The beta cells of your pancreas make insulin and release it in pulses in response to your most recent meal. Its job at those moments is to get the excess nutrients out of your bloodstream so they can be stored for future use. Fat goes into fat cells, protein into muscle cells, and glucose into the liver or muscles, where it's converted to glycogen, or to the fat cells, where it's used for energy or converted to fat. Insulin also *prevents* those tissues from releasing their stored nutrients, which makes perfect sense. So fat stays in fat cells, protein and glycogen stay in muscle cells, and glycogen stays in the liver.

When your body no longer produces enough insulin, one of the first signs is that you lose a lot of weight without trying. You can't get nutrients into cells, and you can't prevent the nutrients already in cells from leaving. Blood sugar climbs so high that you eventually enter a state of glucotoxicity, literally poisoning yourself with your own blood. The damage to your beta cells can be permanent if it isn't reversed in time.

In that situation, your doctor will immediately and aggressively use an insulin medication to bring your blood sugar down and save your pancreas, if not your life. But in the absence of glucotoxic symptoms—excessive thirst and copious urination, in addition to unexplained weight loss—I almost always try other approaches before considering insulin.

Many doctors would tell you there's a firm line dividing those who need to start taking insulin and those who can try other therapies first. Let's say, for example, that you walk into the doctor's office with an A1C approaching 10 percent. (As you may recall, 6.5 percent is the borderline for diabetes.) Some doctors would start insulin therapy immediately. I prefer to see what the patient is willing to do with diet, exercise, and one or more of the medications I described in the previous sections. I would run out of fingers counting the patients who came to me with an A1C of 12 percent who brought their blood sugar down without insulin. That's partly because the other medications are really good, and partly because the patients bought into the lifestyle changes I discussed with them.

I don't say that to make you feel bad if you need insulin, now or in the future. I just want you to know there's a lot you can do short of taking it.

## Starting Insulin Therapy

In a nonemergency situation, I'll start a patient with insulin if the other measures don't bring her A1C down to her target level. Those targets will differ from one patient to the next. Patients who are older (65 plus) and have had type 2 diabetes longer (10 years or more) will have a higher target. Those who are younger, newly diagnosed, and actively trying to get leaner and healthier will have a lower, more aggressive target.

We start with a *basal insulin*. These are insulin analogs—genetically engineered to have a long-lasting effect—that you inject once a day, usually with dinner or before bed. I like to start with detemir (Levemir) because it's associated with less weight gain. Others prefer glargine (Lantus), which is also taken once a day, either in the morning or at night. Glargine seems to have a longer-lasting effect than detemir. There's also a newer drug called degludec (Tresiba) that lasts even longer. All of them were developed as improvements on NPH (Humulin), a synthetic version of human insulin. NPH is an intermediate-acting drug, lasting about 10 to 16 hours, as opposed to 24 hours for the basal insulins.

Insulin therapy puts a lot of responsibility on the patient in the beginning. After she takes her injections at night, she has to check her own blood sugar the next morning. If it's 130 or higher for a couple of mornings in a row (we want to see fasting glucose below 100), she'll have to *titrate*—that is, slowly increase her own dose every few days, based on her doctor's instructions.

Conversely, if she experiences hypoglycemia, and her fasting blood glucose is below 70, then she and her doctor will have to adjust her medications, her diet, or both.

Some patients also require prandial insulin—a fast-acting insulin taken with a meal. Your doctor may prescribe lispro (Humalog), aspart (NovoLog), or glulisine (Apidra). When and how often these are used will vary from patient to patient. We also have the option of using two types of insulin simultaneously, either premixed or with separate injections.

## Short-Term Insulin Therapy

Some doctors will use insulin right away with newly diagnosed type 2 patients, even in nonemergency situations. The rationale is that it gives the pancreas a reboot, allowing it to take a breather while the medicine takes blood sugar down to the target level. At that point the pancreas has fully recovered and is newly able to release an appropriate amount of insulin in response to normal meals.

In theory, and I guess in practice in some controlled studies, it allows patients to control their blood sugar without medication . . . assuming those patients also modify their diets and increase their physical activity.

So why don't I use this approach? Because if I can get patients to eat better and move more, we can achieve the same result without insulin, and without the risk of hypoglycemia and weight gain.

## WEIGHT-LOSS MEDICATIONS

You know I'm a strong advocate of nutrition, exercise, and lifestyle as the first line of defense against obesity, diabetes, heart disease, and countless other problems. So when I talk about drugs that help my patients lose weight, I expect to get some pushback. It seems like a blatant contradiction. But it's not. If a patient is trying to stick to a sensible diet but can't control her cravings, I can use one of these four medications. They aren't "fat-burning" pills. They work either by reducing appetite, and thus taking the edge off those cravings, or by preventing food from being fully absorbed during the digestive process. The downside is that most people regain the weight if they stop using the medications.

# INSULIN FOR LIFE? NOT NECESSARILY!

Sometimes my patients amaze me. Take Doris. At 65, she was taking two types of insulin—a long-acting daily injection (what we call a basal insulin) and smaller, fast-acting doses with meals. I didn't think we'd be able to get her off insulin entirely, but since she was motivated to change her lifestyle, I hoped we could at least eliminate the need for the mealtime injections.

We accomplished that goal with some dietary adjustments and post-meal walks. What surprised me is that we also reduced the need for basal insulin while still controlling her blood sugar. It was a longer process, but with the combination of her new diet, daily exercise, and about 15 to 20 pounds of weight loss, she finally got off insulin altogether.

I wouldn't say Doris reversed her diabetes entirely—she still takes two medications—but she feels much better now and is happy that she no longer needs those daily insulin shots.

Dave faced a very different challenge. He was 52 and had recently undergone gastric bypass surgery. But the surgery didn't work the way he expected. He was still taking massive amounts of insulin, which was delivered through a pump because his blood sugar was so poorly controlled he couldn't risk waiting for a daily injection.

I knew he couldn't manage his blood sugar until he lost weight. He couldn't lose weight until he got off insulin. But without insulin, how would he manage his blood sugar?

Fortunately, he was willing to make two big changes: He switched to my version of the Mediterranean diet, with lower carbohydrates and higher protein. And he also walked a lot, every day. His adherence to those changes allowed us to stop his insulin while substituting two drugs that make it easier to lose weight.

His blood sugar went up at first, as I feared, but Dave's dedication to the diet and exercise program made the new program work. He has lost 60 pounds so far and doesn't need insulin anymore.

Phentermine/topiramate extended release (Qsymia) combines two strange bed-fellows. Phentermine was once partnered with fenfluramine in a notorious weight-loss drug called fen-phen. It was eventually linked to potentially fatal cardiovascular problems, became the subject of billions of dollars' worth of lawsuits in the 1990s, and was taken off the market. On its own, though, phentermine was first approved in 1959 as an obesity treatment, and it has a long track record as an effective short-term appetite suppressant.

## DANGER ZONES

We've focused on the inner workings of type 2 diabetes—how it affects your blood sugar, and how various hormones respond, or fail to respond. But if you have diabetes, you also have external challenges. The longer you've had it, especially if it went untreated for a while, the more damage will accrue to your nerves and blood vessels, especially in your feet and eyes.

### Feet

**The problem:** The heavier you are, the older you are, and the longer you've had diabetes, the greater the risk there is to your feet. Nerve damage can make you insensitive to open sores or infections that would have driven your younger self up a wall. Circulation damage prevents the normal healing process from taking place. Your weight and lack of flexibility prevent you from being able to see the damage, especially when it's on the bottom of your feet or between your toes.

**Your job:** Your doctor should examine your feet during regular appointments. In between those checkups, you have to find a way to see what's going on at ground level. If you can't get a family member or close acquaintance to help, you need to do it yourself, using mirrors if necessary.

**Watch out for:** Even if you can't feel the tips of your toes or bottoms of your feet, you should notice any change in your balance or stride.

Topiramate is an anticonvulsant that's also been used to control migraines. The two medications work on different parts of the brain to reduce appetite and can safely be used for long-term weight control. I've seen dramatic weight loss in some of my patients, along with drops in blood sugar and blood pressure.

The biggest risk is birth defects. If you're female, fertile, and sexually active, you *must* use contraception while taking it, and should also do a pregnancy test every month, just to be safe.

**Pro move:** You can head off some of the nerve and circulation problems with simple foot exercises. For example, you can sit in a chair and then crab-walk your toes across a carpeted floor by flexing and relaxing them. Or you can fill a baking dish with sand (or fresh cat litter) and practice squeezing the sand with your toes. (Just make sure you don't have any open cuts or sores before you stick your feet into sand.) These exercises improve circulation while they strengthen the muscles in your feet.

### Eyes

**The problem:** High blood sugar, elevated lipids (LDL and triglycerides), and high blood pressure have the potential to damage the tiny veins and capillaries that keep your eyes healthy and vision strong.

**Your job:** Regular eye exams are a must. An ophthalmologist should be able to detect changes to your vision or anomalies caused by impaired circulation.

**Pro move:** Anything that makes your eyes tired or sore—staring at a computer screen, squinting in bright sunlight, wearing contact lenses for too long—can exacerbate eye problems brought on by diabetes or high blood pressure. Give your eyes regular breaks from the screen, shield them from the sun, and occasionally wear glasses instead of contacts.

Lorcaserin (Belviq) is a serotonin agonist, which means it activates a receptor in your brain that responds to serotonin, a powerful mood-altering hormone. It reduces appetite and may also help lower blood sugar. You have to be extremely cautious about combining it with an antidepressant or any other drug that affects serotonin.

Naltrexone/bupropion extended release (Contrave) combines two drugs used to combat addiction. Bupropion (Wellbutrin) is one of the rare antidepressants that *isn't* linked to weight increases. It's been used successfully to help smokers quit, and may help with amphetamine addiction as well. Naltrexone combats opioid and alcohol dependence. I find this one especially useful for patients who tell me they crave particular foods.

There are two drawbacks. The first is the hassle factor: You have to gradually increase the dosage from one to four pills a day—two in the morning and two in the evening. The other is that naltrexone reverses the effects of opioids, so if you're taking a narcotic, you can't use Contrave.

If orlistat (Xenical or Alli) sounds familiar, it's probably because of its infamous side effects: steatorrhea (the medical term for greasy stools), and fecal discharge when passing gas (a polite way to describe a shart). It works by blocking fat absorption in your digestive tract, which helps you lose weight. But if the fat isn't used for energy, it has to go somewhere else, and you can only hope it's your toilet and not your underwear. The version called Alli is available over the counter in the United States. The more potent Xenical is prescription-only, but as you probably guessed, I don't prescribe it very often.

## CHAPTER 15

# Is Diabetes Ever "Beaten"? It All Depends on Your Point of View

**WHEN YOU GET A COLD OR THE FLU,** you know with almost perfect certainty that you will recover. Even if it isn't much consolation when you're burning up with fever or your sinuses feel like an inflated balloon, it's still something to look forward to.

But is it possible to recover from type 2 diabetes? If you do every single thing I describe in this book—you eat better, exercise consistently, get higher-quality sleep, and lose weight—is there a chance to *beat* diabetes for good?

Here's the honest answer: I don't know.

What I do know, because I've seen it many times, is that some patients can bring their blood sugar back to normal levels and go off medications entirely. Others improve dramatically and get along with just one drug like metformin. They no longer have the primary symptom of type 2 diabetes, which is chronically elevated blood sugar. Everyone who makes a serious, sustained effort to lead a healthier, more active life improves his or her diabetes symptoms in measurable ways.

What I don't know is exactly how to describe the end result. I like to say my most successful patients *reverse* diabetes. At that point they've certainly beaten the disease. Other doctors use more cautious language and say it's in *remission,* rather than saying the patient has recovered. That implies, of course, that the doctor expects diabetes to return, and that the patient should prepare for it.

So which is correct? Is it possible to fully recover from type 2 diabetes, to beat this disease once and for all? Let's take a deeper look.

## THE BEST-CASE SCENARIO

I talked about weight-loss surgery in Chapter 3, and how patients' blood sugar often returns to normal just days after the procedure. Recently, researchers at Newcastle University in England tried to achieve the same results without surgery. They recruited 30 adults with diabetes, most of whom also had obesity, and put them on an extremely low-calorie diet. For 8 weeks the subjects got just 624 calories a day from three Optifast meal-replacement shakes, plus a little more from nonstarchy vegetables. To put that in perspective, for someone eating 3,500 calories a day—a conservative estimate for the heaviest in the study group—that's an 80 percent drop in calories. Imagine doing this for 56 consecutive days without a break.

It did indeed work much like surgery: The average participant lost 35 pounds, and regained only a couple of them over the next 6 months. More important, 12 of the 30 had fasting blood sugar below 126 (the cutoff for diabetes) without medicine, although at an average of 114, they were still in the prediabetic range.

The 12 with the best results were on average younger (early versus late fifties), had a more recent diagnosis (4 versus 10 years), and started the program with lower fasting blood sugar and less total body fat. They were also using fewer medications; in fact, five weren't using any drugs at all.

Here's my point: If we're going to talk about full recovery from type 2 diabetes, we have to start with an honest look at the challenges. Among those whose diabetes is reversed by weight-loss surgery, half eventually become diabetic again. And among those in the Newcastle study who endured an almost impossibly strict diet for 8 weeks, fewer than half saw their fasting blood sugar fall below the cutoff for diabetes.

These data points track pretty well with my own experience. Remember Jason, the patient I described in Chapter 1? He checked a couple of the boxes for someone ideally positioned to reverse his condition. At 45, he was still young for a diabetes patient, and although his blood sugar was sky-high when he came to my office, the fact he hadn't previously been diagnosed worked in his favor. Once he got serious about diet and exercise, he also had the advantage of "newbie gains"—that's what we call it when your body responds right away to a new program. He was motivated, he followed through on my advice, he worked hard, and he soon brought his blood sugar down to normal levels.

Now we return to the semantics of *recovery* or *reversal* versus *remission*. Many doctors and researchers—most, I'd estimate—will say that once you have type 2 diabetes, the conditions are always in place. The best you can hope for is remission, with constant vigilance and effort to keep it from returning.

But we don't really have proof. We can measure blood sugar, of course, and more sophisticated tests can quantify the ability of your pancreas to produce insulin. We can also assess the conditions related to diabetes—waist size, blood pressure, cholesterol and triglyceride levels, liver and kidney function. The one thing we *can't* do is isolate a single causal element, like a virus or bacterium, and tell a patient, "See this squiggly thing? Sorry, that's diabetes."

Without certainty, we're left with two questions: Are you getting better? Or worse?

## THE GREAT UNKNOWN

When I began working with patients who have diabetes, the consensus among my colleagues was that the condition only gets worse. Prediabetes becomes diabetes.

With diabetes comes the need for insulin. With insulin comes further weight gain. Weight gain reduces the patient's physical activity, which was probably limited to begin with, and that makes everything worse. The path isn't necessarily *straight* downhill, but once you start rolling in that direction, you aren't likely to stop. It's similar to the way we approach our aging patients: We expect them to gain weight, to need drugs to control their blood pressure and cholesterol, to become weak and frail.

I've never believed it has to be that way. My time as an athlete, and my lifelong interest in health and fitness, has led me to countless stories of individuals who overcame extraordinary challenges. In my medical practice, I can't say I have *countless* examples of patients reversing diabetes; I'm sure I could count them if I really wanted to. I just know there are a lot. More important, the ones who successfully lowered their blood sugar and regained their health weren't always the ones I would've considered the best candidates—the youngest, lightest, or most recently diagnosed.

My goal, both in these pages and in my practice, is to give encouragement without crossing over into false hope. It's never easy to change our patterns, especially those we consider lifelong, familial, or even multigenerational. The way we eat, the amount of time we spend moving, our sleep habits—all those things make up who we are. It's possible to change them, but they rarely give up without a fight. And yet, some patients do it, with spectacular success. Some struggle and occasionally take a step back, but achieve very good results when they stick to their plan. Others just struggle. And to be frank, some don't even try. They'll let the drugs do the work of controlling their disease.

I don't know where you'll fall on that spectrum. You probably don't know either. Neither of us can predict which bits of advice will resonate, or which interventions will deliver the biggest improvements. One patient of mine lost 20 pounds when he stopped going to McDonald's for lunch every day. (I'm pretty sure that one would work for anybody.) But some of you have already done the obvious things, like not eat fast food seven times a week. The next steps are anything but certain. Nothing works for everyone.

So here's what I can guarantee: If you do what I've covered in this book—if you eat better and lose a few pounds; if you begin and stick with a systematic exercise routine; if you get better sleep; and if you change up your routines to allow those actions and behaviors to become part of your identity—you *will* get better. Your health *will* improve. You *will* have more energy and a greater sense of control.

And, yes, many of you will beat diabetes. For how long, I can't say. It might be a few years, it might be much more. There's only one way to find out.

# More Go-To Meals

**THESE RECIPES** came from Rodale's test kitchen, with ingredients and portions that are more precisely calculated than my own. They're also more complex and labor-intensive than the suggestions in Chapter 11, but they are great options to add to your menus of healthy and delicious meals.

# SOUPS

## CHUNKY TILAPIA AND TOMATO SOUP

**FOR 2 SERVINGS:**

⅓ cup thinly sliced carrots

⅓ cup thinly sliced red onion

1 tablespoon olive oil

½ teaspoon dried thyme

Salt to taste

2 cups chicken broth

1 cup water

12 ounces tilapia fillets, cut into large chunks

1½ cups chopped broccoli florets

1 cup canned diced tomatoes, with juice

½ teaspoon ground black pepper

In a large saucepan, combine the carrots, onion, oil, thyme, and salt to taste. Cook over medium heat, stirring, for 5 minutes, or until softened. Add the broth and water. Bring almost to boiling. Add the tilapia, broccoli, tomatoes, and pepper. Reduce the heat and simmer for 8 minutes, or until the tilapia is cooked.

*Totals (per serving): 319 calories, 42 grams protein, 10 net grams carbs (14 grams carbs, 4 grams fiber), 11 grams fat*

# COCONUT-LIME SHRIMP SOUP

4 carrots, cut into matchsticks

3 heads baby bok choy, sliced

1 clove garlic, minced

1 tablespoon grated fresh ginger

2 cups chicken broth

1 can (13.5–14 ounces) light coconut milk

1 cup water

2 teaspoons soy sauce

½ teaspoon red or green curry paste

4 ounces multigrain or whole wheat angel hair pasta, broken in half

1 pound large shrimp, peeled and deveined

2 tablespoons lime juice

1. Coat a large saucepan with cooking spray and heat over medium heat. Add the carrots, bok choy, garlic, and ginger and cook, stirring, for 3 minutes, or until fragrant. Add the broth, coconut milk, water, soy sauce, and curry paste. Increase the heat to medium-high and cook just until the mixture comes to a boil.

2. Add the pasta. Bring to a boil, then reduce the heat to medium and simmer for 4 minutes, or until the pasta is almost tender.

3. Stir in the shrimp. Cook for 1 to 3 minutes, or until the shrimp are opaque and the pasta is tender. Remove from the heat and stir in the lime juice.

*Totals (per serving): 366 calories, 32 grams protein, 26 net grams carbs (33 grams carbs, 7 grams fiber), 13 grams fat*

# TRADITIONAL BEEF-BARLEY SOUP

**FOR 4 SERVINGS:**

⅓ cup unbleached all-purpose flour

1 pound beef stew meat, cubed

2 tablespoons olive oil

8 ounces mushrooms, thinly sliced (about 2 cups)

2 onions, finely chopped

1 rib celery, finely chopped

2 cups beef broth

2 cups water

3 tablespoons barley

1 carrot, finely chopped

1 bay leaf

2 teaspoons chopped fresh thyme or 1 teaspoon dried

½ teaspoon ground black pepper

1 tablespoon soy sauce

1. Place the flour in a resealable plastic bag. Add the beef, seal the bag, and toss to coat.

2. In a large saucepan over medium-high heat, heat the oil. Add the beef and cook, stirring frequently, for 8 minutes, or until browned. Add the mushrooms, onions, and celery. Cook, stirring occasionally, for 7 minutes, or until the mushrooms and onions are lightly browned.

3. Stir in the broth, water, barley, carrot, bay leaf, thyme, pepper, and soy sauce. Bring to a boil. Reduce the heat to low, cover, and simmer for 2 hours, or until the beef and barley are tender. Discard the bay leaf.

*Totals (per serving): 444 calories, 42 grams protein, 22 net grams carbs (26 grams carbs, 4 grams fiber), 19 grams fat*

# SALADS

## STEAK WITH BULGUR SALAD

**FOR 4 SERVINGS:**

1 cup bulgur (cracked wheat)

1 cup boiling water

4 tomatoes, each cut into 8 wedges

2 tablespoons chopped red onion

¼ cup red wine vinegar

2 tablespoons olive oil

5 radishes, sliced

1 cucumber, sliced

1 cup fresh parsley, chopped

¼ teaspoon ground black pepper

¾ teaspoon salt, divided

1 pound sirloin steak, trimmed of visible fat

1. Place the bulgur in a medium bowl. Cover with the boiling water. Fluff with a fork and let sit for 10 minutes, or until the water is absorbed.

2. Meanwhile, in a large bowl, combine the tomatoes, onion, vinegar, oil, radishes, cucumber, parsley, pepper, and ½ teaspoon of the salt. Once the bulgur is ready, gently stir it into the tomato mixture.

3. Coat a skillet with cooking spray and heat over medium heat. Sprinkle the steak with the remaining ¼ teaspoon salt and cook, turning once, for 6 to 8 minutes, or until a thermometer inserted in the center registers 145°F for medium-rare. Transfer the steak to a cutting board and let it rest for 10 minutes. Then slice the steak and place it over the salad.

*Totals (per serving): 402 calories, 31 grams protein, 31 net grams carbs (40 grams carbs, 9 grams fiber), 13 grams fat*

# BEEF AND VEGGIE SALAD BOWL

FOR 1 SERVING:

3 ounces lean beef, cubed

2 tablespoons dry red quinoa

2 teaspoons olive oil

1 teaspoon red wine vinegar

2 cups mesclun greens

½ cup chopped broccoli florets

¼ red bell pepper, chopped

1. Preheat the broiler. Coat the broiler pan rack with cooking spray.

2. Broil the beef cubes until cooked through.

3. Prepare the quinoa according to package directions.

4. *To make the dressing:* In a small bowl, whisk the oil and vinegar together. When the steak and quinoa are cooked, combine them in a bowl with the greens, broccoli, and pepper. Add the dressing and toss to coat.

*Totals: 353 calories, 31 grams protein, 16 net grams carbs (21 grams carbs, 5 grams fiber), 17 grams fat*

*Recipe courtesy of Keri Glassman*

# LUNCHES AND DINNERS

## CHILI-SPICED TURKEY-BEAN BURGERS WITH GUACAMOLE

**FOR 4 SERVINGS:**

**GUACAMOLE**

1 ripe avocado, halved, pitted, and peeled

2 tablespoons chopped sweet white onion

1 tablespoon salsa

1 tablespoon lime juice

**BURGERS**

⅔ cup canned black beans, rinsed and drained

1 pound lean ground turkey breast

1 egg

2 teaspoons chili powder

½ teaspoon ground cumin

½ teaspoon salt

Whole grain hamburger buns

Tomato slices

1. *To make the guacamole:* In a small bowl, mash the avocado with a fork until fairly smooth. Mix in the onion, salsa, and lime juice. Cover tightly and set aside.

2. *To make the burgers:* Preheat the broiler. Coat the broiler pan rack with cooking spray. In a medium bowl, mash the beans to a chunky texture. Stir in the turkey, egg, chili powder, cumin, and salt until well blended. Shape into 4 burgers.

3. Broil the patties 4" to 6" from the heat for 12 minutes, turning once, or until a thermometer inserted in the center registers 160°F and the meat is no longer pink. Place on a plate.

4. Toast the buns on the broiler pan until lightly browned. Serve the burgers on the buns with a tomato slice and guacamole.

> *Totals: 386 calories, 38 grams protein, 26 net grams carbs (37 grams carbs, 11 grams fiber), 13 grams fat*

# LIME-MARINATED CHICKEN WITH SALSA

4 boneless, skinless chicken breasts

3 tablespoons lime juice

2 tablespoons olive oil

1¼ teaspoons ground cumin

¼ teaspoon kosher salt

3 medium tomatoes, chopped

½ avocado, halved, pitted, peeled, and chopped

½ cup chopped sweet onion, such as Vidalia

½ cup chopped cilantro

1 small jalapeño chile pepper, seeded and finely chopped (wear plastic gloves when handling)

4 sprigs cilantro for garnish

4 lime wedges for garnish

1. Put chicken into a large resealable plastic bag. In a small bowl, whisk together the lime juice, oil, cumin, and salt. Transfer 2 tablespoons of the lime marinade to a medium glass bowl for the salsa, and cover with plastic wrap. Pour the remaining marinade over the chicken and squeeze it around to make sure the chicken is fully coated. Let the chicken marinate in the fridge for at least 1 hour.

2. Preheat the broiler and coat the broiler pan rack with cooking spray. Broil the chicken for 13 minutes, turning once, or until a thermometer inserted in the thickest portion registers 165°F and the juices run clear.

3. While the chicken cooks, add the tomatoes, avocado, onion, cilantro, and pepper to the bowl with the reserved marinade. Gently toss to mix. Serve the chicken topped with the salsa and garnished with the cilantro and lime wedges.

*Totals (per serving): 292 calories, 35 grams protein, 6.5 net grams carbs (10 grams carbs, 3.5 grams fiber), 13 grams fat*

# GRILLED TUNA STEAKS
# TOPPED WITH LEMONY ARTICHOKE HEARTS

**FOR 4 SERVINGS:**

1 cup water

¾ cup couscous

4 teaspoons extra-virgin olive oil, divided

12 ounces frozen artichoke hearts, thawed

1 medium onion, chopped

½ teaspoon dried basil

3 cloves garlic, minced

2 teaspoons fresh lemon juice

¼ teaspoon salt, divided

¼ teaspoon ground black pepper, divided

4 yellowfin tuna steaks (4 ounces each)

1 teaspoon ground coriander

1. In a small saucepan over medium-high heat, bring the water to a boil. Stir in the couscous, cover, and remove from the heat. Let stand for 5 minutes and then fluff with a fork. Keep warm.

2. In a large nonstick skillet over medium-high heat, heat 3 teaspoons of the oil. Cook the artichokes, onion, and basil for 5 minutes, stirring occasionally, or until the artichokes are browned. Add the garlic and cook for 4 minutes, or until the onion is lightly browned. Stir in the lemon juice and cook for 30 seconds. Remove from the heat and stir in ⅛ teaspoon of the salt and ⅛ teaspoon of the pepper. Keep warm.

3. Coat a grill pan with cooking spray and heat over medium-high heat. Rub the tuna with the remaining 1 teaspoon oil. Sprinkle with the coriander and the remaining ⅛ teaspoon salt and pepper. Cook the tuna for 8 minutes, turning once, or until the fish is just opaque. Serve with the couscous and artichokes.

*Totals (per serving): 310 calories, 32 grams protein, 22 net grams carbs (29 grams carbs, 7 grams fiber), 6 grams fat*

# SEARED SNAPPER
## ON HERBED AND MASHED EDAMAME

**FOR 4 SERVINGS:**

2 cups frozen shelled edamame

4 shallots, finely chopped

½ teaspoon dried tarragon

1½ cups water

1 tablespoon lemon juice

1½ pounds snapper, cod, or haddock fillets, cut into 4 pieces

½ teaspoon salt

½ teaspoon ground black pepper

1. In a small saucepan, combine the edamame, shallots, tarragon, and water. Bring to a boil over high heat. Reduce the heat to low, cover, and simmer for 20 minutes, or until very tender. Transfer to a blender or food processor and blend until smooth, adding the lemon juice and a little water if needed. Return to the saucepan, cover, and keep warm.

2. Sprinkle the fish with the salt and pepper. Coat a large nonstick skillet with cooking spray and heat over medium-high heat. Cook the fish, turning once, for 8 to 10 minutes, or until it flakes easily.

3. Serve the fish on top of the edamame mixture.

*Totals (per serving): 279 calories, 43 grams protein, 7 net grams carbs (11 grams carbs, 4 grams fiber), 5 grams fat*

# Pork Chops Baked with Cabbage and Cream

**FOR 4 SERVINGS:**

1 small head (1½ pounds) green cabbage, cored and finely shredded

4 boneless pork chops (6 ounces each), each ¾" thick

½ teaspoon salt, divided

¼ teaspoon ground black pepper

2 teaspoons olive oil

½ cup half-and-half

1 teaspoon caraway seeds

½ teaspoon sweet Hungarian paprika

1 teaspoon dried marjoram or thyme

½ cup (2 ounces) shredded Swiss cheese

1. Preheat the oven to 350°F.

2. Bring a large pot of salted water to a boil over high heat. Add the cabbage and cook for 4 to 5 minutes, or until soft. Drain in a colander and dry it well with paper towels.

3. Season the pork chops with ¼ teaspoon of the salt and the pepper. In a large, heavy, ovenproof skillet over high heat, heat the oil. Cook the pork chops for 1 to 2 minutes, turning once, or just until browned. Remove to a plate.

4. Discard any fat in the skillet and heat over low heat. Stir in the cabbage, half-and-half, caraway seeds, paprika, marjoram or thyme, and the remaining ¼ teaspoon salt. Cook and stir until heated through, about 1 minute. Remove from the heat and arrange the pork over the cabbage, adding any juices accumulated on the plate. Sprinkle with the cheese. Bake for 25 minutes, or until a thermometer inserted in the center of a chop registers 145°F.

*Totals (per serving): 413 calories, 45 grams protein, 8 net grams carbs (13 grams carbs, 5 grams fiber), 20 grams fat*

# GRILLED STEAK AND WARM BEAN SALAD

**FOR 4 SERVINGS:**

3 tablespoons balsamic vinegar, divided

1 clove garlic, lightly mashed

1¼ pounds flank steak

   Salt to taste

   Ground black pepper to taste

1 can (16 ounces) cannellini beans, rinsed and drained

1 cup cherry tomatoes, halved

½ cup thinly sliced red onion

1 tablespoon extra-virgin olive oil

1 large bunch arugula, stems trimmed

1. Pour 2 tablespoons of the vinegar into a baking dish. Rub the garlic all over the steak, put the steak into the dish, and turn to coat both sides with the vinegar. Cover and refrigerate for 30 to 60 minutes to 1 hour.

2. Heat a large nonstick grill pan over medium-high heat. Remove the steak from the marinade and pat dry. Sprinkle with salt and pepper to taste. Grill the steak for 5 to 7 minutes, or until browned on both sides and a thermometer inserted in the center registers 145°F for medium-rare.

3. In a saucepan or a microwaveable bowl, heat the beans. Stir in the tomatoes, onion, oil, remaining 1 tablespoon vinegar, and salt and pepper to taste. Mix well.

4. Cut the steak into thin slices and serve it over the arugula, alongside the salad.

*Totals (per serving): 368 calories, 36 grams protein, 17 net grams carbs (23 grams carbs, 6 grams fiber), 14 grams fat*

# ITALIAN SEAFOOD STEW

**FOR 4 SERVINGS:**

1 tablespoon olive oil

1 medium bulb fennel, chopped (reserve the fronds)

1 onion, chopped

4 cloves garlic, roughly chopped

½ teaspoon fennel seeds

½ teaspoon red-pepper flakes

1 can (28 ounces) whole peeled tomatoes

12 ounces clam juice

1 cup chicken stock

1½ cups red wine (pinot noir)

2 bay leaves

½ teaspoon dried thyme

Salt to taste

Ground black pepper to taste

1 pound firm white fish, such as halibut or cod, cut into chunks

½ pound medium shrimp, peeled and deveined

12–16 mussels, scrubbed and debearded

1. In a large saucepan or pot over medium heat, heat the oil. Add the fennel, onion, garlic, fennel seeds, and red-pepper flakes and cook, stirring, until the vegetables are soft, about 5 minutes.

2. Lightly crush the tomatoes with your fingers (careful: juice may splatter from inside them) and discard the remaining tomato juice from the can. Add the tomatoes to the pan, along with the clam juice, chicken stock, wine, bay leaves, and thyme, and bring to a simmer. Cook for 5 minutes, taste, and adjust the seasoning with salt and black pepper.

3. Place the fish, shrimp, and mussels in the pan. Cook for 5 minutes, or until the fish is firm, the shrimp are pink, and the mussels are open. Discard the bay leaves. Serve with the reserved fennel fronds for garnish.

*Totals (per serving): 499 calories, 36 grams protein, 18 net grams carbs (23 grams carbs, 5 grams fiber), 22.5 grams fat*

# Beef and Black Bean Chili

1 tablespoon olive oil

1½ pounds lean ground beef

2 red onions, cut into thin wedges

3 cloves garlic, minced

1 can (15 ounces) crushed tomatoes

2 jalapeño chile peppers, seeded and chopped (wear plastic gloves when handling)

1 tablespoon chili powder

1 teaspoon cumin seeds

1 teaspoon dried oregano

½ teaspoon sugar

¼ teaspoon celery seeds

1 tomato, chopped

2 cans (15 ounces each) black beans, rinsed and drained

1. In a large saucepan over medium-high heat, heat the oil. Cook the beef, stirring frequently, for 8 minutes, or until no longer pink. Add the onions and cook, stirring occasionally, for 5 minutes, or until softened. Add the garlic and cook for 1 minute.

2. Add the crushed tomatoes, peppers, chili powder, cumin seeds, oregano, sugar, and celery seeds. Bring to a boil. Reduce the heat to low, cover, and simmer for 10 minutes. Add the chopped tomato and beans. Cook for 3 minutes to heat through.

*Totals (per serving): 336 calories, 34 grams protein, 23 net grams carbs (33 grams carbs, 10 grams fiber), 9 grams fat*

# CHICKEN PHO WITH BUCKWHEAT NOODLES

**FOR 4 SERVINGS:**

- 4 ounces buckwheat (soba) noodles
- 12 ounces chicken tenders, cut into thin strips
- 4 cups chicken broth
- 8 baby bok choy, quartered lengthwise
- ½ cup shelled edamame
- ½ red bell pepper, cut into thin strips
- 1 small bunch scallions, sliced
- 1 teaspoon toasted sesame oil
- 1 teaspoon soy sauce
- ½ cup fresh cilantro, coarsely chopped
- 1 lime, cut into wedges

1. Prepare the noodles according to package directions, but cook for about 4 minutes (or 1 minute less than directed on the package). Drain well.

2. Meanwhile, coat a saucepan with cooking spray and heat over medium-high heat. Cook the chicken, stirring, for 4 minutes, or until browned. Add the broth and bring to a boil. Add the bok choy and edamame and simmer for 4 minutes, or until the chicken is cooked through.

3. Stir in the pepper and scallions. Cook for 2 minutes. Remove from the heat and stir in the sesame oil, soy sauce, and cilantro. Divide the noodles among 4 soup bowls. Pour the chicken mixture over the noodles. Serve with the lime wedges.

*Totals (per serving): 272 calories, 30 grams protein, 27 net grams carbs (31 grams carbs, 4 grams fiber), 4 grams fat*

# Glazed Salmon with Broiled Pineapple Slaw

**FOR 4 SERVINGS:**

4 salmon fillets (5 ounces each)

½ cup pineapple chunks

1 tablespoon lime juice

1 tablespoon honey

1½ cups thinly sliced cabbage

1 carrot, grated

1 tablespoon roasted or raw sunflower seeds

1 tablespoon chopped fresh cilantro

1. Preheat the broiler. Line the rack of a broiler pan with foil and coat with cooking spray. Arrange the salmon and pineapple on the foil. In a small bowl, combine the lime juice and honey. Drizzle 2 teaspoons over the salmon and pineapple. Set aside the remaining lime juice mixture.

2. Broil the salmon and pineapple for 6 to 7 minutes, or just until the fish is opaque and the pineapple is lightly browned.

3. Meanwhile, in a large bowl, combine the cabbage, carrot, sunflower seeds, and cilantro. Add the broiled pineapple to the cabbage mixture and toss with the reserved lime juice mixture. Serve the fish with the slaw on the side.

*Totals (per serving): 350 calories, 30 grams protein, 9 net grams carbs (11 grams carbs, 2 grams fiber), 20 grams fat*

# Rosemary Lamb Stew

**FOR 6 SERVINGS:**

1½ tablespoons olive oil

1½ tablespoons butter

3 pounds lamb, fat removed, cut into 1½" cubes

½ teaspoon dried rosemary

2 cloves garlic, mashed

½ teaspoon ground black pepper

1 tablespoon unbleached all-purpose flour

¾ cup red wine

1 cup chicken stock

4 anchovy fillets, mashed

Parsley sprigs for garnish

3 cups cooked brown rice (optional)

1. In a Dutch oven (or deep ovenproof skillet or soup pot) over medium-high heat, heat the oil and butter. Cook the lamb, stirring, for 5 minutes or until browned. Add the rosemary, garlic, and pepper.

2. In a small bowl, blend the flour with a little of the wine to form a paste, then add the rest of the wine to the paste and stir to combine. Add to the lamb.

3. Add the stock and cook, stirring, until slightly thickened. Cover and simmer for 1 hour, stirring from time to time, or until the meat is tender.

4. Dip out ½ cup of the sauce and transfer to a small bowl. Add the anchovies and stir to combine. Pour the mixture back into the stew and stir to blend. Simmer for 5 minutes, garnish with parsley, and serve either by itself or with brown rice.

*Totals (per serving): 412 calories, 48 grams protein, 3.5 net grams carbs (no fiber), 19 grams fat*

*Totals (per serving, with ½ cup cooked brown rice): 521 calories, 50 grams protein, 23 net grams carbs (25 grams carbs, 2 grams fiber), 20 grams fat*

# MOROCCAN STEWED CHICKEN

**FOR 4 SERVINGS:**

½ tablespoon olive oil

1 pound boneless, skinless chicken thighs

Salt to taste

Ground black pepper to taste

1 large zucchini, cut into cubes

1 can (16 ounces) chickpeas, rinsed and drained

1 can (14.5 ounces) diced tomatoes, with juices

1 cup chicken stock or water

½ teaspoon ground red pepper

1 teaspoon ground cumin

½ teaspoon ground cinnamon

¼ cup chopped cilantro

1. In a large skillet or wide pot over medium-high heat, heat the oil.

2. Season the chicken with salt and black pepper to taste and cook for 4 to 6 minutes, turning once, or until browned. Add the zucchini and cook, stirring often, until the zucchini has browned lightly.

3. Add the chickpeas, tomatoes and juice, chicken stock or water, red pepper, cumin, and cinnamon. Reduce the heat to low and simmer for 10 to 15 minutes, or until the chicken is tender and a thermometer inserted in the center of a thigh registers 165°F. Season to taste with additional salt and black pepper. Garnish with the chopped cilantro.

*Totals (per serving): 373 calories, 30 grams protein, 27 net grams carbs (34 grams carbs, 7 grams fiber), 12 grams fat*

# SPICED BEEF AND LENTIL STEW

1 tablespoon olive oil

1 large onion, sliced

4 cloves garlic, minced

1 teaspoon paprika

½ teaspoon dried thyme

½ teaspoon ground cumin

¼ teaspoon salt

½ teaspoon ground black pepper

⅛ teaspoon ground allspice

⅛ teaspoon ground red pepper

1 pound lean, well-trimmed boneless beef chuck, cut into ½" cubes

2 tablespoons unbleached all-purpose flour

1½ cups chicken broth

¾ cup water

¾ cup lentils, picked over and rinsed

2 large carrots, sliced

1. Preheat the oven to 325°F. In a Dutch oven (or deep ovenproof skillet or soup pot) over medium heat, heat the oil. Add the onion and garlic and cook, stirring often, for 5 minutes, or until tender (add a tablespoon of water if the pan gets dry). Stir in the paprika, thyme, cumin, salt, black pepper, allspice, and red pepper. Cook and stir for 1 minute.

2. On a plate, toss the beef with the flour. Add the floured beef to the pot and stir to coat well with the spices and onion. Pour in the broth and water and bring to a boil.

3. Cover and transfer to the oven. Bake for 45 minutes, or until the meat starts to get tender. Add the lentils and carrots; cover and bake for 40 to 50 minutes, or until the beef and lentils are tender.

*Totals (per serving): 327 calories, 31 grams protein, 21 net grams carbs (34 grams carbs, 13 grams fiber), 7.5 grams fat*

# Sample Meal Plans

There is no simple way to estimate exactly how much food any individual should eat for any particular goal. Your age, gender, diet, body composition (percentage of fat versus lean tissue), activity level, and health status all factor in. The online calculator I mentioned earlier (niddk.nih.gov/health-information/health-topics /weight-control/body-weight-planner/pages/bwp.aspx) gives you a pretty good estimate of how much you eat now to maintain your current weight.

But to lose weight? That's trickier. Success depends on adherence. Adherence depends on sustainability. Sustainability depends on how well the new, lower-calorie diet fits into your life. Do you like the food? How much time and energy do you have to put into the shopping and meal prep? Can you go at least 4 hours between meals without feeling so hungry it becomes a distraction?

Those questions aren't quite as important at the beginning, when you're changing your habits, developing a new roster of go-to meals, and adjusting to less food. You need a reasonably high level of motivation and commitment to get through the initial inconvenience and discomfort. But if the pieces don't feel like they're falling into place, you aren't likely to stick with it long enough to get the results you want.

With that out of the way, let's look at three sample plans. Most are based on the go-to meals from Chapter 11, although you'll also see a few from Appendix A. Total calories average about 1,500 a day in the first plan, which would be appropriate for an older, less active female, or someone who's ready for an aggressive weight-loss plan. The second offers about 1,900 calories a day, and the third weighs in at just under 2,300 a day. (The average is 2,258.)

Protein ranges from about 25 to 35 percent of total calories, with total carbs usually below 30 percent. That's fewer carbs than most of my patients are used to, but not what the purists I know would consider a genuine low-carb diet. (While there isn't a *strict* definition, anything greater than 20 percent of daily calories would be outside of their parameters.)

Each plan includes 5 days' worth of meals. Following these guidelines for 2 or 3 weeks can help you adjust to your new diet. But remember: It's just a sample of how you can eat. You can dive into the plan as it's laid out, or just use it as a template for building your own menu—by following the overarching guidelines on pages 118 to 119. Stick to those, first and foremost, and you should have great success. Below is a little more background on the plan.

A few more notes about my thought process.

- You'll see some repetition in the breakfast choices, since most of us eat more or less the same things for breakfast each day. If you *literally* have the same thing every day, adjust the plan accordingly.

- The two higher-calorie plans include a daily smoothie, where you'll also see some repetition—once again, because that's what people who have daily protein shakes seem to do.

- I include leftovers at least once in each plan. It's usually a lunch made from the previous night's dinner. If that's not appealing to you, switch the leftovers out for something in the same calorie range.

- Finally, I put in a glass of wine with each dinner in the first two plans, and two glasses with dinner in the highest-calorie plan. If you prefer something else, you can make a one-for-one exchange of a beer or mixed drink. And if you don't drink at all, you can either save the calories or substitute a piece of fruit.

# PLAN ONE: ABOUT 1,500 CALORIES A DAY

| DAY 1 | | |
|---|---|---|
| Breakfast | Lunch | Dinner |
| High-Protein Oatmeal with Chia Seeds (page 121) | Caprese Salad (page 127) | Roast Chicken with Sweet Potatoes and Red Wine (page 129); side salad; glass of red wine |
| *Totals:* 1,450 calories, 92 grams protein, 69.5 net grams carbs (89 grams carbs, 19.5 grams fiber), 72.5 grams fat | | |

| DAY 2 | | |
|---|---|---|
| Breakfast | Lunch | Dinner |
| Crabby Eggs (page 122) | Turkey Sandwich with Avocado (page 123) | Baked Salmon with Green Beans (simple version) (page 130); side salad; glass of white wine |
| *Totals:* 1,508 calories, 115 grams protein, 65 net grams carbs (88 grams carbs, 23 grams fiber), 63 grams fat | | |

| DAY 3 | | |
|---|---|---|
| Breakfast | Lunch | Dinner |
| High-Protein Oatmeal with Chia Seeds (page 121) | Totally Not from the Mediterranean Burrito Bowl (page 126) | Roast Chicken with Sweet Potatoes and Red Wine (leftovers); side salad; glass of red wine |
| *Totals:* 1,515 calories, 106.5 grams protein, 100.5 net grams carbs (128 grams carbs, 27.5 grams fiber), 54.5 grams fat | | |

| DAY 4 | | |
|---|---|---|
| Breakfast | Lunch | Dinner |
| Cottage Cheese with Fruit and Nuts (using 1% fat cottage cheese) (page 121) | Turkey Sandwich with Avocado (page 123) | Beef and Veggie Salad Bowl (page 240); side salad; glass of red wine |

*Totals:* 1,469 calories, 102 grams protein, 60 net grams carbs (88 grams carbs, 28 grams fiber), 68 grams fat

| DAY 5 | | |
|---|---|---|
| Breakfast | Lunch | Dinner |
| High-Protein Oatmeal with Chia Seeds (page 121) | Greek Tuna Salad (page 126) | Chili-Spiced Turkey-Bean Burgers with Guacamole (page 241); side salad; glass of white wine |

*Totals:* 1,497 calories, 101.5 grams protein, 78.5 net grams carbs (110.5 grams carbs, 32 grams fiber), 62 grams fat

# PLAN TWO: ABOUT 1,900 CALORIES A DAY

| DAY 1 | | | |
|---|---|---|---|
| Breakfast | Lunch | Snack | Dinner |
| Cottage Cheese with Fruit and Nuts (page 121) | Turkey Sandwich with Avocado (page 123) | Every Day's a Holiday smoothie (page 132) | Baked Salmon with Green Beans (with pistachios) (page 130) and a glass of white wine |

*Totals:* 1,905 calories, 150 grams protein, 100 net grams carbs (132 grams carbs, 32 grams fiber), 74.5 grams fat

| DAY 2 | | | |
|---|---|---|---|
| Breakfast | Lunch | Snack | Dinner |
| No-Brainer Eggs (page 121) | Greek Tuna Salad (page 126) | Smoothie Bowl (page 133) | Steak, Hold the Potatoes (page 127), and a glass of red wine |

*Totals:* 1,884 calories, 131.5 grams protein, 77.5 net grams carbs (102.5 grams carbs, 25 grams fiber), 89.5 grams fat

| DAY 3 | | | |
|---|---|---|---|
| Breakfast | Lunch | Snack | Dinner |
| Breakfast Burrito (page 122) | Greek Tuna Salad (leftovers) | ¼ cup cashews | Super-Simple Slow-Cooked Chicken Chili (page 128); side salad; glass of white wine |

*Totals:* 1,902 calories, 142.5 grams protein, 82.5 net grams carbs (106.5 grams carbs, 24 grams fiber), 87.5 grams fat

| DAY 4 | | | |
|---|---|---|---|
| Breakfast | Lunch | Snack | Dinner |
| Cottage Cheese with Fruit and Nuts (page 121) | Super-Simple Slow-Cooked Chicken Chili (leftovers) | The Breakfast Date smoothie (page 132) | Beef and Veggie Salad Bowl (page 240) and a glass of red wine |

*Totals:* 1,871 calories, 160 grams protein, 94 net grams carbs (122 grams carbs, 28 grams fiber), 73 grams fat

| DAY 5 | | | |
|---|---|---|---|
| Breakfast | Lunch | Snack | Dinner |
| Breakfast Burrito (page 122) | Big Salad (page 123) | The Starter Kit smoothie (page 131) | Super-Simple Slow-Cooked Chicken Chili (leftovers) and a glass of white wine |

*Totals:* 1,862 calories, 169 grams protein, 70 net grams carbs (98 grams carbs, 28 grams fiber), 84.5 grams fat

# PLAN THREE: ABOUT 2,300 CALORIES A DAY

| DAY 1 | | | |
|---|---|---|---|
| Breakfast | Lunch | Snack | Dinner |
| Cheese and Veggie Omelet (page 122) | Big Salad (page 123) | Smoothie Bowl (page 133) | Super-Simple Slow-Cooked Chicken Chili (page 130); side salad; 2 glasses of white wine |

*Totals:* 2,261 calories, 164 grams protein, 88 net grams carbs (123 grams carbs, 35 grams fiber), 99 grams fat

| DAY 2 | | | |
|---|---|---|---|
| Breakfast | Lunch | Snack | Dinner |
| Breakfast Burrito (page 122) | Super-Simple Slow-Cooked Chicken Chili (leftovers) | Every Day's a Holiday smoothie (page 132) | Steak, Hold the Potatoes (page 127); side salad; 2 glasses of red wine |

*Totals:* 2,296 calories, 173 grams protein, 108 net grams carbs (135 grams carbs, 27 grams fiber), 96 grams fat

| DAY 3 | | | |
|---|---|---|---|
| Breakfast | Lunch | Snack | Dinner |
| Cottage Cheese with Fruit and Nuts (page 121) | Greek Tuna Salad (page 126) | Smoothie Bowl (page 133) | Baked Salmon with Green Beans (with pistachios) (page 130); side salad; 2 glasses of white wine |

*Totals:* 2,259 calories, 147.5 grams protein, 90.5 net grams carbs (130.5 grams carbs, 40 grams fiber), 97 grams fat

| DAY 4 | | | |
|---|---|---|---|
| Breakfast | Lunch | Snack | Dinner |
| Cheese and Veggie Omelet (page 122) | Greek Tuna Salad (leftovers) | Every Day's a Holiday smoothie (page 132) | Roast Chicken with Sweet Potatoes and Red Wine (page 129); side salad; 2 glasses of red wine |

*Totals:* 2,217 calories, 131.5 grams protein, 109.5 net grams carbs (136.5 grams carbs, 27 grams fiber), 96 grams fat

| DAY 5 | | | |
|---|---|---|---|
| Breakfast | Lunch | Snack | Dinner |
| Cottage Cheese with Fruit and Nuts (page 121) | Roast Chicken with Sweet Potatoes and Red Wine (leftovers) | Smoothie Bowl (page 133) | Lime-Marinated Chicken with Salsa, 2 portions (page 242); side salad; 2 glasses of white wine |

*Totals:* 2,259 calories, 168 grams protein, 85 net grams carbs (121 grams carbs, 36 grams fiber), 99 grams fat

# RESOURCES

## More from the Author

**My blog:** drspencer.com

Social media:

- Facebook: Dr. Spencer Nadolsky (facebook.com/DrSpencerNadolsky)
- Twitter: @DrNadolsky

**My first book:** *The Fat Loss Prescription: The Nine-Step Plan for Losing Weight and Keeping It Off* (available at amazon.com or drspencer.com)

## Books about Food, Habits, and Weight Loss

**How our food chain got so messed up:** *The End of Overeating,* by David A. Kessler, MD (Rodale, 2010).

**Habits and behaviors:** *Mindless Eating: Why We Eat More Than We Think* (Bantam, 2006) and *Slim by Design: Mindless Eating Solutions for Everyday Life* (William Morrow, 2014), by Brian Wansink, PhD.

**Health and weight management:** *Eat Well, Move Well, Live Well: 52 Ways to Feel Better in a Week,* by Roland Denzel and Galina Denzel (with a foreword by me) (Propriometrics Press, 2016).

**Weight control and body composition (emphasis on muscle development):** *The Lean Muscle Diet,* by Lou Schuler and Alan Aragon (Rodale, 2014).

## Books about Fitness and Strength Training

**For older, heavier, and/or nontraditional lifters:** *The New Rules of Lifting for Life: An All-New Muscle-Building, Fat-Blasting Plan for Men and Women Who Want to Ace Their Midlife Exams,* by Lou Schuler and Alwyn Cosgrove (Avery, 2012).

**Lower-back health and core training:** *Back Mechanic: The Secrets to a Healthy Spine Your Doctor Isn't Telling You,* by Stuart McGill, PhD (Backfitpro, 2015).

**Interval training:** *The One-Minute Workout,* by Martin Gibala, PhD, with Christopher Shulgan (Avery, 2017).

## Online Programs and Apps

**For novice runners:** I highly recommend Couch to 5K (C25K), which is available free at coolrunning.com (and many other sites). It was invented by Josh Clark, a software designer, in 1996. He says that most users will be able to jog 3 miles nonstop by the end of the 9-week program. You can buy his C25K apps for $1.99 at iTunes and Google Play.

**For weight management:** Myfitnesspal.com is a popular site with free tracking tools for your daily meals. I recommend it to almost all of my patients, and many have used it with great success.

**For better sleep:** Myshuti.com offers cognitive behavioral therapy for insomnia (CBT-I). You'll need to invest some time (about an hour a week) and a little money ($135 for a 16-week subscription when we went to press), but it's been worth the cost for the patients who've gone through the program.

# REFERENCES

## Introduction

***"Eat less, move more":*** "Weight Loss Doctor Says 'Eat Less, Move More' Is Awful Advice," by Lou Schuler (menshealth .com, August 24, 2015).

## Chapter 1

***Dr. Google:*** Yes, we typed "blurred vision excessive urination" into the search engine, and the first two links had "diabetes symptoms" in the title.

***Diabetes prevalence:*** US estimates are from "Statistics about Diabetes," by the American Diabetes Association (diabetes.org/diabetes-basics/statistics). International numbers are from "Global Report on Diabetes" (World Health Organization, April 2016).

## Chapter 2

***Development of medical insulin:*** "The History of Insulin," by Deepinder Brar (med.uni-giessen.de/itr/history/inshist .html).

***Risk factors:*** The statistics I used are from the US Centers for Disease Control and Prevention (cdc.gov/diabetes/data /index.html).

***Mitochondria:*** *The New Rules of Lifting for Life,* by Lou Schuler and Alwyn Cosgrove (Avery, 2012), pp. 15–17; Kitt Falk Petersen et al., "Mitochondrial dysfunction in the elderly: possible role of insulin resistance," *Science* 2003; 300 (5622): 1140–42; Ian R. Lanza and K. Sreekumaran Nair, "Mitochondrial function as a determinant of life span," *European Journal of Physiology* 2010; 459: 277–89.

***BMI and diabetes:*** Michael L. Ganz et al., "The association of body mass index with the risk of type 2 diabetes: a case-control study nested in an electronic health records system in the United States." *Diabetology & Metabolic Syndrome* 2014; 6: 50.

***Waist-to-height ratio:*** Satoru Kodama et al., "Comparisons of the strength of associations with future type 2 diabetes risk among anthropometric obesity indicators, including waist-to-height ratio: a meta-analysis." *American Journal of Epidemiology* 2012; 176 (11): 959–69; "Waist to Height Ratio (WHtR)," by Penn State PRO Wellness (prowellness .vmhost.psu.edu/prevention/understanding_risk/whtr).

***Blood sugar:*** *Molecular Biology of the Cell,* Fourth Edition, by Bruce Alberts et al. (Garland Science, 2002), pp. 103–4; Chris Masterjohn, "Sugar Is the Ultimate Antioxidant and Insulin Will Make You Younger," *Examine.com Research Digest* 2016; 19 (1): 12–15.

## Chapter 3

***Fat-generated hormones:*** Erin E. Kershaw and Jeffrey S. Flier, "Adipose tissue as an endocrine organ." *The Journal of Clinical Endocrinology & Metabolism* 2004; 89 (6): 2548–66; Kathryn A. Britton and Caroline S. Fox, "Ectopic fat depots and cardiovascular disease." *Circulation* 2011; 124: e837–41; Aurelie Villaret et al., "Adipose tissue endothelial cells from obese human subjects: differences among depots in angiogenic, metabolic, and inflammatory gene expression and cellular senescence." *Diabetes* 2010; 59: 2755–63; David E. Kelley and Bret H. Goodpaster, "Stewing in not-so-good juices: interactions of skeletal muscle with adipose secretions." *Diabetes* 2015; 64: 3055–57; Vanessa Pellegrinelli et al., "Human adipocytes induce inflammation and atrophy in muscle cells during obesity." *Diabetes* 2015; 64: 3121–34.

***Look AHEAD study:*** Rena R. Wing et al., "Benefits of modest weight loss in improving cardiovascular risk factors in overweight and obese individuals with type 2 diabetes." *Diabetes Care* 2011; 34: 1481–86; Thomas A. Wadden et al., "Four-year weight losses in the Look AHEAD study: factors associated with long-term success." *Obesity* 2011; 19 (10): 1987–98; The Look AHEAD Research Group, "Eight-year weight losses with an intensive lifestyle intervention: the Look AHEAD study." *Obesity* 2014; 22 (1): 5–13.

***Weight loss of more or less than 5 percent:*** Marion J. Franz et al., "Lifestyle weight-loss intervention outcomes in overweight and obese adults with type 2 diabetes: a systematic review and meta-analysis of randomized clinical trials." *Journal of the Academy of Nutrition and Dietetics* 2015; 115: 1447–63.

***Weight-loss surgery:*** Francesco Rubino et al., "Metabolic surgery in the treatment algorithm for type 2 diabetes: a joint statement by international diabetes organizations." *Diabetes Care* 2016; 39 (6): 861–77; Andrei Keidar, "Bariatric surgery for type 2 diabetes reversal: the risks." *Diabetes Care* 2011; 34 (Supplement 2): S361–S266.

***Fat loss in liver and pancreas:*** This comes from research by Roy Taylor, MD, and his team at Newcastle University's Magnetic Resonance Centre in the UK. See the notes for Chapter 15.

***Weight-loss success:*** "I'm an Obesity Doctor. I've Seen Long-Term Weight Loss Work. Here's How," by Yoni Freedhoff (vox.com, May 10, 2016).

***Rate of weight loss:*** Krista Casazza et al., "Myths, presumptions, and facts about obesity." *New England Journal of Medicine* 2013; 368: 446–54.

## Chapter 4

***Exercise guidelines:*** Sheri R. Colberg et al., "Exercise and type 2 diabetes." *Diabetes Care* 2010; 33 (12): 2692–96.

***Exercise versus diabetes:*** "Exercise: The Miracle Cure and the Role of the Doctor in Promoting It," by the Academy of Medical Royal Colleges (aomrc.org.uk, 2015).

***Minimal amount of exercise:*** Paddy C. Dempsey et al., "Benefits for type 2 diabetes of interrupting prolonged sitting with brief bouts of light walking or simple resistance activities." *Diabetes Care* 2016; 39 (6): 964–72.

***Cardio versus strength training:*** Timothy S. Church et al., "Effects of aerobic and resistance training on hemoglobin A1C levels in patients with type 2 diabetes." *Journal of the American Medical Association* 2010; 304 (20): 2253–62; Zuyao Yang et al., "Resistance exercise versus aerobic exercise for type 2 diabetes: a systematic review and meta-analysis." *Sports Medicine* 2014; 44: 487–99.

***Muscle quality:*** Martin Sénéchal et al., "Association between changes in muscle quality with exercise training and changes in cardiorespiratory fitness measures in individuals with type 2 diabetes mellitus: results from the HART-D Study." *PLoS One* 2015; 10 (8): e0135057.

***Weight loss variability:*** Neil A. King et al., "Individual variability following 12 weeks of supervised exercise: identification and characterization of compensation for exercise-induced weight loss." *International Journal of Obesity* 2008; 32 (1): 177–84.

## Chapter 5

***Sleep, obesity, and diabetes:*** Eliane A. Lucassen et al., "Interacting epidemics? Sleep curtailment, insulin resistance, and obesity." *Annals of the New York Academy of Sciences* 2012; 1264: 110–34; "Sleep Matters for Obesity," by Karl Nadolsky and Spencer Nadolsky (medpagetoday.com, November 20, 2015).

***Purpose of sleep:*** "What You Should Know about Sleep," by Chad Waterbury (chadwaterbury.com, May 6, 2016); "The Benefits of Slumber: Why You Need a Good Night's Sleep" (*NIH News in Health,* April 2013).

***Sleep and Alzheimer's:*** Lulu Xie et al., "Sleep drives metabolite clearance from the adult brain." *Science* 2013; 342 (6156): 373–77; "Lack of Deep Sleep May Set the Stage for Alzheimer's," by Jon Hamilton (npr.org, January 4, 2016).

***Sleep apnea:*** "Tired All the Time? Snore? Check for Sleep Apnea," by Spencer Nadolsky (drspencer.com); Paul E. Peppard et al., "Increased prevalence of sleep-disordered breathing in adults." *American Journal of Epidemiology* 2013; 177 (9): 1006–14.

**Weight loss:** Hutan Ashrafian et al., "Bariatric surgery or non-surgical weight loss for obstructive sleep apnea? A systematic review and comparison of meta-analyses." *Obesity Surgery* 2015; 25 (7): 1239–50; Lana J. Mitchell et al., "Weight loss from lifestyle interventions and severity of sleep apnea: a systematic review and meta-analysis." *Sleep Medicine* 2014; 15 (10): 1173–83; Anil Anandam et al., "Effects of dietary weight loss on obstructive sleep apnea: a meta-analysis." *Sleep and Breathing* 2013; 17 (1): 227–34.

**Light exposure:** Kenji Obayashi et al., "Ambient light exposure and changes in obesity parameters: a longitudinal study of the HEIJO-KYO cohort." *Journal of Clinical Endocrinology & Metabolism* 2016: jc20154123.

**Diphenhydramine danger:** Shelly L. Gray et al., "Cumulative use of strong anticholinergics and incident dementia." *JAMA Internal Medicine* 2015; 175 (3): 401–7.

**Allergy pills and weight gain:** Joseph C. Ratliff et al., "Association of prescription H1 antihistamine use with obesity: results from the National Health and Nutrition Examination Survey." *Obesity* 2010; 18 (12): 2398–400.

**Cognitive behavioral therapy for sleep:** "Sleep like a Baby: Myths about Insomnia and Aging," by Stanford Hospital Health Library (shlnews.org, January 28, 2016).

**Sleep myths:** Tero Myllymaki et al., "Effects of vigorous late-night exercise on sleep quality and cardiac autonomic activity." *Journal of Sleep Research* 2011; 20 (1, Part 2): 146–53; "Unleash the Power of the Nap," by Brett and Kate McKay (artofmanliness.com, February 7, 2011); "21 Health Benefits of Napping," by Korin Miller (menshealth.com, May 27, 2015); "Can Exercising at Night Hurt Your Sleep?" by Tom DiChiara (upwave.com, April 22, 2014).

## Chapter 6

**Metabolism:** Anja Bosy-Westphal el al., "Contribution of individual organ mass loss to weight loss-associated decline in resting energy expenditure." *American Journal of Clinical Nutrition* 2009; 90 (4): 993–1001; Dympna Gallagher et al., "Small organs with a high metabolic rate explain lower resting energy expenditure in African American than in white adults." *American Journal of Clinical Nutrition* 2006; 83 (5): 1062–67; "Most of Us Misunderstand Metabolism. Here Are 9 Facts to Clear That Up," by Julia Belluz (vox.com, May 18, 2016); "BMR versus RMR," by April Merritt (acefitness.org, April 12, 2010).

**Willie Sutton:** Sutton robbed a lot of banks, but according to David Mikkelson at snopes.com, he never said he did it "because that's where the money is." He credited the phrase to "some enterprising reporter who apparently felt a need to fill out his copy." Despite its shaky origins, the phrase was adapted as Sutton's Law, which, in medicine, says that you should always start with the obvious when diagnosing a patient. Don't go full *House* until you've ruled out the likeliest cause, using the simplest and most reliable tests. As a trouble-shooting maxim, it can also be applied to diet and weight loss, telling you not to do the more severe and drastic interventions until you've tried the simple and obvious—like the ones described in Chapter 6.

**Post-meal walk:** "Really? The Claim: Taking a Walk after a Meal Aids Digestion," by Anahad O'Connor (nytimes.com, June 24, 2013).

**Brian Wansink:** *Mindless Eating: Why We Eat More Than We Think* (Bantam, 2006), and *Slim by Design: Mindless Eating Solutions for Everyday Life* (William Morrow, 2014).

## Chapter 7

**Comparing diets:** Amir Emadian et al., "The effect of macronutrients on glycemic control: a systematic review of dietary randomized controlled trials in overweight and obese adults with type 2 diabetes in which there was no difference in weight loss between treatment groups." *British Journal of Nutrition* 2015; 114: 1656–66.

**Honey and hunter-gatherers:** "The *Real* Paleo Diet," by Lou Schuler and John Williams, PhD (menshealth.com, November 1, 2013).

**Glycemic index and glycemic load:** "The Truth about the Glycemic Index," edited by Alan Aragon (menshealth.com, October 14, 2013).

***Fiber versus diabetes:*** Robert E. Post et al., "Dietary fiber for the treatment of type 2 diabetes mellitus: a meta-analysis." *Journal of the American Board of Family Medicine* 2012; 25: 16–23; James W. Anderson et al., "Health benefits of dietary fiber." *Nutrition Reviews* 2009; 67 (4): 188–205.

***Whole grains:*** Dagfinn Aune et al., "Whole grain consumption and risk of cardiovascular disease, cancer, and all cause mortality: systematic review and dose-response meta-analysis of prospective studies." *BMJ* 2016; 353: i2716.

***Alcohol history:*** "How to Eat Like a Caveman (the Real Kind)," by John Williams (louschuler.com, November 6, 2013).

***Alcohol, health, and weight control:*** "Does Booze Have Metabolic Merits?" by Karl Nadolsky and Spencer Nadolsky (medpagetoday.com, March 30, 2016); "Which Alcohol Should You Drink for Weight Loss?" by Spencer Nadolsky (drspencer.com).

***Alcohol and diabetes:*** Xiao-Hua Lie et al., "Association between alcohol consumption and the risk of incident type 2 diabetes: a systematic review and dose-response meta-analysis." *American Journal of Clinical Nutrition* 2016; 103: 818–29; Yftach Gepner et al., "Effects of initiating moderate alcohol intake on cardiometabolic risk in adults with type 2 diabetes." *Annals of Internal Medicine* 2015; 163: 569–79.

## Chapter 8

***Protein used for energy:*** *Dietary Protein and Resistance Exercise,* edited by Lonnie Lowery and Jose Antonio (CRC Press, 2012), p. 4.

***Protein and diabetes:*** Stuart M. Phillips et al., "Protein 'requirements' beyond the RDA: implications for optimizing health." *Applied Physiology, Nutrition, and Metabolism* 2016; 41: 565–72; Amy Y. Liu et al., "Prevention of type 2 diabetes through lifestyle modification: Is there a role for higher-protein diets?" *Advances in Nutrition* 2015; 6: 665–73.

***Types of protein and diabetes risk:*** Vasanti S. Malik et al., "Dietary protein intake and risk of type 2 diabetes in U.S. men and women." *American Journal of Epidemiology* 2016; 183 (8): 715–28; An Pan et al., "Red meat consumption and risk of type 2 diabetes: three cohorts of U.S. adults and an updated meta-analysis." *American Journal of Clinical Nutrition* 2011; 94 (4): 1088–96.

## Chapter 9

***Ancient humans:*** "How to Eat Like a Caveman (the Real Kind)," previously cited.

***Fat in the American diet:*** "Dietary Intake for Adults 20 Years of Age and Over," National Center for Health Statistics (cdc.gov/nchs/fastats/diet.htm).

***Ancel Keys:*** You can find a terrific summary of Keys's work at sevencountriesstudy.com/home. For more on low-fat dieting, see "The History of Diet Books," by Lou Schuler (menshealth.com, December 31, 2014).

***Flawed premise:*** Zoe Harcombe et al., "Evidence from randomized controlled trials did not support the introduction of dietary fat guidelines in 1977 and 1983: a systematic review and meta-analysis." *Open Heart* 2015; 2: e000196; Russell J. de Souza et al., "Intake of saturated and trans unsaturated fatty acids and risks of all-cause mortality, cardiovascular disease, and type 2 diabetes: systematic review and meta-analysis of observational studies." *BMJ* 2015; 351: h3978; Katherine Keyes and Sandro Galea, "What matters most: quantifying an epidemiology of consequence." *Annals of Epidemiology* 2015; 25 (5): 305–11.

***Milk fat:*** Helena Lindmark Mansson, "Fatty acids in bovine milk fat." *Food & Nutrition Research* 2008; 52.

***Monounsaturated fats and diabetes:*** Lukas Schwingshackl and Georg Hoffmann, "Monounsaturated fatty acids and risk of cardiovascular disease: synopsis of the evidence available from systematic reviews and meta-analyses." *Nutrients* 2012; 4 (12): 1989–2007.

***Nuts and weight:*** Chandra L. Jackson and Frank B. Hu, "Long-term associations of nut consumption with body weight and obesity." *American Journal of Clinical Nutrition* 2014; 100 (Supplement 1): 408S–11S.

# Chapter 10

**Benefits of diet:** Katherine Esposito et al., "A journey into the Mediterranean diet and type 2 diabetes: a systematic review with meta-analysis." *BMJ Open* 2015; 5: e008222.

**Risks of an unhealthy diet:** U.S. Burden of Disease Collaborators, "The state of U.S. health, 1990-2010: burden of diseases, injuries, and risk factors." *Journal of the American Medical Association* 2013; 310 (6): 591–606.

**Thirty percent protein reduces appetite:** Eveline A. Martens et al., "Protein leverage effects of beef protein on energy intake in humans." *American Journal of Clinical Nutrition* 2014; 99 (6): 1397–406.

**Ketogenic diet:** Richard D. Feinman et al., "Dietary carbohydrate restriction as the first approach in diabetes management: critical review and evidence base." *Nutrition* 2015; 31: 1–13.

**Meal replacements:** Thomas A. Wadden et al., "One-year weight losses in the Look AHEAD study: factors associated with success." *Obesity* 2009; 17 (4): 713–22; Linda E. Mignone et al., "Whey protein: the 'whey' forward for treatment of type 2 diabetes?" *World Journal of Diabetes* 2015; 6 (14): 1274–84; Guido Camps et al., "Empty calories and phantom fullness: a randomized trial studying the relative effects of energy density and viscosity on gastric emptying determined by MRI and satiety." *American Journal of Clinical Nutrition* 2016; doi: 10.3945/ajcn.115.129064.

**Satiety index:** Susanna H. Holt et al., "A satiety index of common foods." *European Journal of Clinical Nutrition* 1995; 49 (9): 675–90.

**Insulin index:** Susanna H. Holt et al., "An insulin index of foods: the insulin demand generated by 1,000 kilojoule [239 calorie] portions of common foods." *American Journal of Clinical Nutrition* 1997; 66 (5): 1264–76.

# Chapter 11

**Bread history:** I found the story I relate at foodtimeline.org/foodsandwiches.html. The historical account is attributed to *Encyclopedia of Food and Culture,* Volume 3, edited by Solomon H. Katz (Charles Scribner's Sons, 2003).

**Colt revolver:** You've probably heard some variation on this saying: "God created men, but Sam Colt made them equal." Ironically, Colonel Samuel Colt didn't live long enough to witness the outsize role his namesake pistols (including one called the Peacemaker) would have in westward expansion. If he had any interest in leveling the playing field, it was by selling arms to both sides in various conflicts, including the American Civil War. He was just 47 when he died of gout in 1862, barely a year into the war.

**Estimating portion sizes:** Several tips came from this article: "Twelve Easy Ways to Estimate Serving Sizes," by the editors of *Men's Health* (menshealth.com, April 6, 2015).

# Chapter 12

**"Big Three" stability exercises:** *Back Mechanic,* by Stuart McGill (Backfitpro.com, 2015), pp. 101–9.

# Chapter 13

**METs and longevity:** Scott Trappe et al., "New records in aerobic power among octogenarian lifelong endurance athletes." *Journal of Applied Physiology* 2013; 114: 3–10; Haitham M. Ahmed et al., "Maximal exercise testing variables and 10-year survival: fitness risk derivation from the FIT Project." *Mayo Clinic Proceedings* 2015; 90 (3): 346–55.

**MET values of various activities:** Like calorie counts, these come from a variety of sources, starting with this one: Barbara E. Ainsworth et al., "Compendium of physical activities: an update of activity codes and MET intensities." *Medicine & Science in Sports & Exercise* 2000; 32 (9 supplement): S498–504.

**Interval training:** Martin J. Gibala et al., "Physiological adaptations to low-volume, high-intensity interval training in health and disease." *Journal of Physiology* 2012; 590 (5): 1077–84.

**Snow shoveling fatalities:** Barry A. Franklin et al., "Snow shoveling: a trigger for acute myocardial infarction and sudden coronary death." *American Journal of Cardiology* 1996; 77 (10): 855–58; Rajesh Janardhanan et al., "The snow shoveler's ST elevation myocardial infarction." *American Journal of Cardiology* 2010; 106 (4): 596–600; "Here's Why Some People Drop Dead While Shoveling Snow," by Brady Dennis (washingtonpost.com, January 21, 2016).

**Strength and longevity:** Darryl P. Leong et al., "Prognostic value of grip strength: findings from the Prospective Urban Rural Epidemiology (PURE) study." *Lancet* 2015; 386 (9990): 266–73; Jonatan R. Ruiz et al., "Association between muscular strength and mortality in men: prospective cohort study." *BMJ* 2008; 337: a439.

**Split routines:** Brad J. Schoenfeld et al., "Influence of resistance training frequency on muscular adaptations in well-trained men." *Journal of Strength and Conditioning Research* 2015; 29 (7): 1821–29; "Bro-Split vs. Total-Body Training: Which Builds More Muscle?" by Brad Schoenfeld (lookgreatnaked.com, July 17, 2015).

**Strength training volume:** Brad J. Schoenfeld et al., "Dose-response relationship between weekly resistance training volume and increases in muscle mass: a systematic review and meta-analysis." *Journal of Sports Sciences* 2016; 19: 1–10; "How Many Sets Do You Need to Perform to Maximize Muscle Gains?" by Brad Schoenfeld (lookgreatnaked .com, July 25, 2016).

## Chapter 14

**Metformin:** "Drug Discovery: Metformin and the Control of Diabetes," by Alan Dronsfield and Pete Ellis (*Education in Chemistry*, November 2011); "Metformin May Have Broad Utility in Cancer," by Sunita Patterson (*OncoLog*, November-December 2014); "Anti-Aging Pill Pushed as Bona Fide Drug," by Erika Check Hayden (nature.com, June 17, 2015).

**Empagliflozin:** Bernard Zinman et al., "Empagliflozin, cardiovascular outcomes, and mortality in type 2 diabetes." *New England Journal of Medicine* 2015; 373: 2117–28.

**Drug recommendations:** Alan J. Garber et al., "Consensus statement by the American Association of Clinical Endocrinologists and American College of Endocrinology on the comprehensive type 2 diabetes management algorithm—2016 executive summary." *Endocrine Practice* 2016; 22 (1): 84–113; Martin J. Abrahamson et al., "AACE/ ACE comprehensive diabetes management algorithm 2015." *Endocrine Practice* 2015; 21 (4): e1–e10.

**Insulin and weight changes:** Jean-Francois Yale et al., "Initiation of once-daily insulin detemir is not associated with weight gain in patients with type 2 diabetes mellitus: results from an observational study." *Diabetology & Metabolic Syndrome* 2013; 5: 56; Sanjoy K. Paul et al., "Weight gain in insulin treated patients by BMI categories at treatment initiation: new evidence from real-world data in patients with type 2 diabetes." *Diabetes, Obesity and Metabolism* 2016; PMID: 27502528.

**Bromocriptine:** Hanno Pijl et al., "Bromocriptine: a novel approach to the treatment of type 2 diabetes." *Diabetes Care* 2000; 23: 1154–61.

**Weight-loss medications:** I have addressed these in my own media and was quoted about them in several articles, including these two: "The Diet Pills That May Actually Work," by Ali Eaves (menshealth.com, September 21, 2015), and "Cutting Calories? Here Are 8 Strategies to Combat Hunger on a Daily Basis," by Lou Schuler (menshealth.com, May 10, 2016). (The latter originally appeared in the April 2016 issue of *Men's Health* as "How to Be Hungry.")

## Chapter 15

**Newcastle University study:** Sarah Steven et al., "Very-low-calorie diet and six months of weight stability in type 2 diabetes: pathophysiologic changes in responders and nonresponders." *Diabetes Care* 2016; 39 (5): 808–15. A wealth of free information is available at Newcastle University's "Reversing Type 2 Diabetes" page (ncl.ac.uk/magres /research/diabetes/reversal.htm), including studies, media reports, diet plans, and a 1-hour lecture by lead scientist Roy Taylor, MD. You can also find shorter clips of Dr. Taylor's lectures and interviews on YouTube by searching for "Roy Taylor diabetes."

# INDEX

Underscored page references indicate boxed text and tables. **Boldface** references indicate photographs.

Legumes. *See also* Beans; Lentils
    fiber-rich, <u>76</u>
    in Mediterranean-based diet,
        105
    as protein source, 82, 87
    types of, 69
Lentils
    Spiced Beef and Lentil Stew,
        253
Leptin, 22–23, 43
Levemir, 223
Lifestyle management, for
        diabetes treatment, vii,
        viii, ix, 4
Light exposure, effect on sleep,
        47–48
Linagliptin, 220
Lipoproteins, 90, 91
Liraglutide, 219
Lispro, 224
Liver
    fatty, 22, 23
    glucose storage in, 10–11
    glycogen storage in, 18, 32, 222
    insulin needed by, 11
Longevity, strength increasing,
        185–87
Lorcaserin, 228
Low-carb diets, 18, 65–66, 77, 78,
        <u>110–11</u>
Low-fat diets, <u>91</u>, 94, 101
Lunches, 123
    Beef and Black Bean Chili, 248
    Big Salad, 123
    Caprese Salad, 127
    Chicken Pho with Buckwheat
        Noodles, 249
    Chili-Spiced Turkey-Bean
        Burgers with Guacamole,
        241
    Glazed Salmon with Broiled
        Pineapple Slaw, 250
    Greek Tuna Salad, 126
    Grilled Steak and Warm Bean
        Salad, 246
    Grilled Tuna Steaks Topped
        with Lemony Artichoke
        Hearts, 243
    Italian Seafood Stew, 247

Lime-Marinated Chicken with
        Salsa, 242
    Moroccan Stewed Chicken, 252
    Pork Chops Baked with
        Cabbage and Cream, 245
    protein sources for, 84
    Rosemary Lamb Stew, 251
    in sample meal plans, <u>256–61</u>
    sandwiches for, <u>124–25</u>
    Seared Snapper on Herbed and
        Mashed Edamame, 244
    Spiced Beef and Lentil Stew,
        253
    Totally Not from the
        Mediterranean Burrito
        Bowl, 126
    Turkey Sandwich with
        Avocado, 123

# M

Macronutrients, 109–12. *See also*
        Carbohydrates; Fats,
        dietary; Protein
Maturity-onset diabetes of the
        young (MODY), <u>17</u>
McGill, Stuart, 168
Meal frequency, 106–7
Meal plans, sample, 255
    1,500-calorie, <u>256–57</u>
    1,900-calorie, <u>258–59</u>
    2,300-calorie, <u>260–61</u>
Meal-replacement smoothies,
        113–16, 131–33
Meats. *See also specific meats*
    portion size of, <u>137</u>
    red, 86–87
Medications
    cost of, <u>217</u>
    diabetes, ix, 6, 216, 218–24, 232
        as adjunct treatment, 218
        reducing or discontinuing,
        viii, 8, 229
    weight-loss, 224, 226–28
Mediterranean diet, <u>27</u>, 78, 101–2,
        105–6
Metabolic equivalent task. *See*
        MET values
Metabolism
    basics of, <u>59</u>

    exercise elevating, 31
    muscle and organs driving,
        58–59
Metformin, 218–19, 221, 228
MET values
    of common activities, 181,
        <u>182–83</u>
    how to increase, 184
Miglitol, 220
Milk fat, 90
Mitochondrial dysfunction, 12
MODY, <u>17</u>
Monogenic diabetes, <u>16–17</u>
Monunsaturated fat, 92, <u>96</u>,
    96–97
Muscle. *See also* Lean mass
    for diabetes prevention, <u>7</u>
    energy from, 60
    glucose storage in, 10
    glycogen storage in, 18, 32, 222
    insulin needed by, 11
    insulin resistance and, 23
    protein for building, 79, 81
Muscle loss
    with age, 12, 81–82
    from crash diets, <u>26</u>
    as diabetes risk factor, 12
    with weight loss, 60
Muscle quality, 33, 35
Myths
    diabetes-related, <u>7</u>
    exercise-related, <u>36–37</u>
    sleep-related, <u>50–51</u>
    weight-loss, <u>26–27</u>

# N

Naltrexone, 228
Naps, benefits of, <u>50–51</u>
Nateglinide, 221
"Natural," meanings of, viii
NDM, <u>17</u>
Neck circumference, sleep apnea
    and, 44
Neonatal diabetes mellitus
    (NDM), <u>17</u>
Nephropathy, 19
Nerve damage, 18
Nesina, 220
Net carbs, 71, 72, 118